Praise for *The Sugar Brain Fix*

"Sugar isn't just bad for your body—it hurts your brain too. Mike's program will walk you through how to kick the sugar and reclaim your brain through a powerful combination of simple behavioral shifts and delicious healing foods."

— **JJ Virgin**, *New York Times* best-selling author, *The Sugar Impact Diet*

"If you feel your brain is out of control you need this book. It is based on science and solid clinical experience. It will help grow your most precious organ—your brain."

— **Daniel Amen, M.D.**, founder of Amen Clinics and *New York Times* best-selling author of *Feel Better Fast and Make It Last*

"Providing the brain with moments of stillness, silence, and serenity are essential in our modern world. Mike's technique is yet another tool to put in your arsenal of clinically validated practices."

— **Dr. Susan Albers, Psy.D.**, *New York Times* best-selling author of *Eat Q* and *50 Ways to Soothe Yourself Without Food*

"Get rid of the toxic gunk that is shrinking your brain. Dr. Mike will help you and your brain glow."

— **Naomi Whittel**, *New York Times* best-selling author of *Glow15*

"Our national addiction to sugar is the basis of much of the chronic disease and poor health in our country. Dr. Mike Dow's revolutionary new book, *The Sugar Brain Fix* combines groundbreaking science with easy-to-implement strategies to help you look and feel your best. A must-read for both doctors and patients everywhere."

— **Anthony Youn, M.D.**, best-selling author of *The Age Fix*

"Sugar is a brain-shrinking, waist-expanding molecule that divorces its whole food source and often couples up with saturated fats (hello, doughnut!), leading to an addictive cycle of eating foods that lack nutritional value, but possess the power to kill: heart disease, stroke, cancer, obesity, and diabetes. As a staunch advocate of whole-food, plant-based eating, I commend Dr. Mike Dow for providing sugar lovers with a program that really works. Of course, I particularly love the vegan options!"

— **Kristi Funk, M.D.**, breast cancer surgeon and best-selling author of *Breast: The Owner's Manual*

"*The Sugar Brain Fix* illuminates the fact that too many American families eat a diet that is not only unhealthy, but hazardous to long-term brain health. This book is a must-read for anyone wanting or needing to improve their nutrition and overall health. Dr. Mike's program will help parents incorporate brain-boosting foods into their everyday diet—which can in turn help them model healthy food habits to their kids—important for everyone's future health!"

— **Tanya Altmann, M.D.**, FAAP, founder of Calabasas Pediatrics Wellness Center and author of *What to Feed Your Baby* and *Baby and Toddler Basics*

"In this brilliant book, Dr. Mike has captured the essential ingredients you can easily implement to bring your brain chemistry back into balance and free you from addictive patterns. With this effective 28-day program, you will detox from the foods that drain your energy and make your brain foggy, while adding activities to enhance your mental clarity and overall vitality. I highly recommend putting this into action today!"

— **Andrea Pennington, M.D.**, founder of In8Vitality and best-selling author of *I Love You, Me!*

"*The Sugar Brain Fix* is a must-read for anyone who wants to keep their brain as healthy as possible while simultaneously trimming their waistline. By helping readers understand which foods to avoid and which foods to embrace, Dr. Dow's 28-day plan will undoubtedly change the lives of people around the world."

— **Nita Landry M.D.**, recurring co-host of the Emmy Award-winning series, *The Doctors*

"Through 20 years of studying the human body, I would consider excess processed sugar and lack of consistent moderate exercise the two biggest health threats in the developed world. Dr. Dow's 'Kediterranean' diet is rock solid nutritionally and has enough flexibility to be used as the foundation for a lifestyle of healthy eating, years beyond the 28-day fix. Additionally, Dr. Dow draws upon years of mental health experience to help the reader find the 'why' of change making, so that they are far more likely to succeed. This book has the power to change lives."

— **Dr. Jedidiah Ballard**, ER physician, former U.S. Army Ranger, and *Men's Health Magazine*, Ultimate Guy

THE

SUGAR BRAIN
FIX

ALSO BY DR. MIKE DOW

Your Subconscious Brain Can Change Your Life: Overcome Obstacles, Heal Your Body, and Reach Any Goal with a Revolutionary Technique*

Chicken Soup for the Soul: Think, Act & Be Happy: How to Use Chicken Soup for the Soul Stories to Train Your Brain to Be Your Own Therapist

Heal Your Drained Brain: Naturally Relieve Anxiety, Combat Insomnia, and Balance Your Brain in Just 14 Days*

Healing the Broken Brain: Leading Experts Answer 100 Questions about Stroke Recovery*

The Brain Fog Fix: Reclaim Your Focus, Memory, and Joy in Just 3 Weeks*

*Available from Hay House
Please visit:

Hay House USA: www.hayhouse.com®
Hay House Australia: www.hayhouse.com.au
Hay House UK: www.hayhouse.co.uk
Hay House India: www.hayhouse.co.in

THE
SUGAR BRAIN
FIX

The 28-Day Plan to Quit Craving the Foods That Are Shrinking Your Brain and Expanding Your Waistline

DR. MIKE DOW

HAY HOUSE, INC.
Carlsbad, California • New York City
London • Sydney • New Delhi

Copyright © 2020 by Dr. Mike Dow Enterprises

Published in the United States by: Hay House, Inc.: www.hayhouse.com® •
Published in Australia by: Hay House Australia Pty. Ltd.: www.hayhouse.com
.au • *Published in the United Kingdom by*: Hay House UK, Ltd.: www.hayhouse
.co.uk • *Published in India by*: Hay House Publishers India: www.hayhouse.co.in

Indexer: J S Editorial, LLC
Cover design: Jason Gabbert
Interior design: Nick C. Welch

Cataloging-in-Publication Data is on file at the Library of Congress.

Hardcover ISBN: 978-1-4019-5666-0
E-book ISBN: 978-1-4019-5667-7
Audiobook ISBN: 978-1-4019-5669-1

10 9 8 7 6 5 4 3 2 1
1st edition, January 2020

Printed in the United States of America

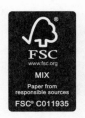
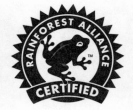

CONTENTS

INTRODUCTION

Sugar: A Codependent Relationship

What's your current relationship status with sugar? If you're like most people today, you'd probably describe it as "in a relationship" or "it's complicated." Sugar is like that bad boyfriend or girlfriend your friends tell you to leave.

Maybe you've tried to leave but have discovered how hard it can be. You still have feelings for sugar. Sugar has always been there for you. It provided comfort when you felt blue. In the best moments of your life, sugar was there to help you celebrate. Maybe you could become "just friends" with sugar—if you could get a little distance from it. But it feels almost impossible. After all, sugar is everywhere.

Perhaps you've tried different strategies to leave this relationship. Maybe you replaced sugar with artificial sweeteners. Or maybe you had no idea you were still eating sugar since the word *sugar* may not be found on the ingredient list. Or you consume foods made from flour and grains—which are then broken down into sugar.

To make matters worse, you've started to hang out with sugar's best buddy: bad fats. Where there's smoke, there's usually fire. And where there's sugar, you can expect to find bad fats. Just about every unhealthy, processed food combines some form of sugar with bad fats. Fats are especially confusing. Which fats are good and which are bad? One day, coconut oil is a good fat. The next day, it's a bad one. At the end of the day, you just end up going back to that ubiquitous combination: sugar with bad fats.

A part of you knows eating this way isn't healthy, but some other part of you rationalizes it. Everyone else is doing it. Eating sugar and bad fats all the time can't be *that* bad, can it? You're not really addicted to it—despite the fact you rarely go a day without foods made from sugar and bad fats. Well, now it's time to face the truth.

I know how you feel, because I used to be in that unhealthy, codependent relationship with sugar. For years, I would drink a daily six-pack of sugar-sweetened soda. The whole experience became a soothing ritual. It began with that piercing pop when I'd open the soda can. Like a Pavlovian dog, I would salivate in anticipation of the serotonin and dopamine hit my brain would soon get from the sugar and caffeine. When I was a teenager, my family would load up on 24-packs from Sam's Club. You could find a reliable stash of at least 50 cans in our house at all times. But my favorite way to get my fix was from fast-food restaurants. I would fill the plastic cup all the way to the top with ice, and, of course, I would refill the cup at least two times. The wide, striped straw of my favorite fast-food restaurant allowed even more of my favorite fix to hit my tongue all at once—a speedball of sugar with a side of stimulant.

While my average intake was six cans during my teens and 20s, bad days would send me bingeing on up to 10 a day. A really bad day at school? Soda's sugar would give me a little soothing serotonin to take the edge off. A boring class? Soda's caffeine would give me the dopamine hit I wasn't getting from a subject I had no interest in. Of course my brain associated it with positive experiences, too. A Friday night or a party would surely mean more soda.

Like many people, I almost always paired my soda with foods made from industrial oils. My after-school snack paired soda with chips or saltines. The weekend party paired soda to wash down pepperoni pizza. Over time, I became addicted to food. And when my brother had a massive stroke when I was in high school, mild self-medication with food turned into all-out binges to deal with the stress and sadness of my family's struggles.

Neurochemically, this isn't surprising. Sugar releases serotonin in the brain, a "feel-good" brain chemical that helps to soothe worries, boost self-confidence, and create a feeling of "okayness" in the world. Bad fats release dopamine, an energizing biochemical we all need to function during stressful situations and exciting challenges. Over time, these sugars and bad fats were shrinking my brain, but the serotonin and dopamine I got from food made this codependent relationship hard to leave.

So I exited this bad relationship with sugars and bad fats but jumped straight into another one. When I moved from Ohio to Los Angeles to attend USC, I noticed a difference in the way people in California ate. It wasn't the meat-and-potatoes diet I was used to in the Midwest, and I was tired of the food coma that came from carb binges. I remember buying a 34-inch-waist pant size—my largest ever—and I knew that something had to change. At the time, I didn't know much about nutrition. So I did what most people did in the early 2000s: I switched to diet soda and diet foods. Low-calorie and low-fat was the name of the game. It was all about *less*. Less sugar. Less fat. Fewer calories. Smaller portions. Downing liters of diet soda every day with reduced-calorie frozen meals became my new norm. It was restriction based with a focus on what I *shouldn't* eat, and while I was consuming fewer brain-shrinking foods, it wasn't really doing much to *grow* my brain.

The Mediterranean Diet and the Brain

Back in 2011, I wrote a book called *Diet Rehab* while hosting a show on TLC called *Freaky Eaters*—where I helped people to break free from their food addictions. That book was based on the research available at the time. The prevailing opinion a decade ago said that cutting calories was the best way to lose weight. Studies showing that the Mediterranean diet can treat depression or that sugar shrinks human brains hadn't been published yet, and *keto* and *paleo* weren't household words.

In the years that followed, I began to read study after study that showed how the Mediterranean diet was absolutely incredible when it came to brain health—while also preventing just about every other major disease. As a brain health expert, I was compelled to change my diet in 2014. At the time, I was researching my book *The Brain Fog Fix*, and every new study I found supported the Mediterranean diet for brain health. And so I began to head in the right direction as I favored foods like fish, olive oil, nuts, and fruit. Finally, I had figured out a way to feel good. Omega-3-rich foods paired with vitamin-rich produce actually helped my brain to manufacture a steady supply of serotonin and dopamine. Everyday choices like exercise also helped me to boost these feel-good neurotransmitters even more.

A few years ago, one study I read took my enthusiasm to a whole new level. It showed that unhealthy food doesn't just mess with your brain chemistry; the damage goes even further. It was the first study that showed *sugar and bad fats can shrink human brains*. As someone who has eaten a lot of sugar and junk food through the years, I knew I needed to fix my own sugar brain. Otherwise, I'd be increasing my risk for depression and dementia. Personally, I want to live a life that's long, healthy, productive, and filled with purpose.

This study also showed that a diet rich in grilled fish and produce was linked to a bigger brain, so the Mediterranean diet I was already following was certainly a step in the right direction. But I wanted to go even further. After all, I had consumed *a lot* of sugar, flour, grains, and bad fats over the years. Soda and boxed macaroni and cheese had been my go-to comfort foods for decades.

To turn things around, I knew I had to create even more brain-derived neurotrophic factor (BDNF), a growth hormone that's often been called Miracle-Gro for the brain. Boosting BDNF is the ultimate antidote for sugar brain. I retained the anti-inflammatory Mediterranean framework, but I began to supercharge it with strategies that would encourage mild ketosis, which helps your body burn stored fat instead of sugar for fuel.

A new diet was emerging.

A Winning Combination: Keto Meets Mediterranean

Ketosis is one of the best ways to boost BDNF levels and also rapidly shed belly fat. Your waistline shrinking is a great indication that your brain is probably growing. Research has proven there's an inverse relationship between belly fat and brain volume. My waistline is now smaller than when I was in my late teens or 20s. I'm thrilled, because I know it's an indication that I'm reversing my own sugar brain—while reducing my risk for just about every major disease.

I used a "Kediterranean"-based (that's what I call ketogenic plus Mediterranean) Sugar Brain Fix. It reverses sugar brain by helping you to grow the same part of the brain that sugar shrinks. The bad news: Sugar brain is real. The good news: Sugar and bad fats shrink a part of the brain that's one of only two places in the brain where new brain cells are created. Translation: Sugar brain is *reversible*.

The Mediterranean framework of my diet takes you back to the diet of Crete, which has been called the original Mediterranean diet. Like vegan and vegetarian diets, it's jam-packed with vegetables and whole fruits that support healthy brain chemistry. In fact, a true Mediterranean diet is often classified as a plant-based diet. Animal protein and dairy are once-in-a-while complements to meals. And when there is a bit of meat, it tends to be high-quality fish. Grass-fed, free-range, and organic animal products have more brain-healthy omega-3s than the factory-farmed varieties with high levels of omega-6s and bad types of saturated fat that are shrinking American brains.

Despite all the other diets that are popular today, the Mediterranean diet still holds its own. In 2019, *U.S. News & World Report* had a large panel of top physicians, dieticians, and researchers evaluate 41 of the most popular diets. The Mediterranean diet was named the number one best diet overall, number one easiest diet to follow, number one best diet for healthy eating, number one best diet for diabetes, number one best heart-healthy diet, and number one best plant-based diet.

The *only* place where the Mediterranean diet *didn't* shine was in the best fast-weight-loss category. Here's where the ketogenic (or keto) diet comes into play. Researchers noted that while keto is extremely hard to follow, it's one of the most effective diets for rapid weight loss. That's important since, as you know, shredding belly fat increases the likelihood you'll have a bigger brain.

By adding just two tools that encourage mild ketosis on top of the Mediterranean framework, you have a winning combination for health, brain growth, *and* shredding belly fat.

The Sugar Brain Fix *Really* Works!

The keto element of this diet takes us back to a time when we were hunters and gatherers—when intermittent fasting and fasted workouts were simply a part of life. Back then, we had to work to find food. Without drive-throughs and 24-hour grocery stores, eating and snacking around the clock wasn't possible. The periods of not having any food would vary from one day to the next, depending on when you could find food that grew in the ground or hunted for it.

As people searched and hunted for food after going variable amounts of time with none, they were actually practicing intermittent fasting. As they chased their prey on an empty stomach, they were doing fasted-state workouts. The diet in this book includes timing workouts with brief fasts, which forces your body to turn to stored fat instead of glucose for fuel. When you do this, you'll still get some of the benefits of longer fasts or strict keto.

Some people wonder if this diet really works. The answer is yes, and throughout this book I'll share some real-life success stories to prove it.

And there's more good news: You can bypass the headaches, constipation, and increased risk of kidney stones that can occur in people doing strict keto with my best-of-both-worlds Kediterranean strategy of the Sugar Brain Fix.

The diet in this book is both fantastic for the brain and easy to follow in the long run. It's much lower in sugars and carbs than the American diet that leads to sugar brain, but not quite as low as a strict keto diet. Grains are drastically reduced but not eliminated—since you can always have a few servings of any type of food you'd like during each week of the 28-day program.

Unlike keto, all whole fruits are encouraged since they're incredible foods for brain health. And there's only one off-limit vegetable: potatoes. (Corn is off-limits if it's processed into chips.) We'll place more emphasis on omega-3-rich proteins, plant-based protein like beans, moderately high good fat, and high levels of antioxidants. In contrast, traditional keto contains high amounts of animal protein and fat, almost no plant-based protein, and relatively lower levels of antioxidants. This is why strict keto leads to an increase in LDL, or "bad," cholesterol in people who follow it. And replacing carbohydrates with high levels of animal protein and low levels of plant-based protein—as people following keto do—has been linked with an increased risk of death.

With its modified approach, this is a middle-of-the-road diet. You can eat both fat and carbs, while reducing sugar, flour, grains, and industrial oils and increasing vegetables, fruit, and olive oil. It's far more complex and nuanced than the black-or-white approach of the nonfat or all-carbs-are-the-devil way of eating. The *type* of carbs and fat matter, because all carbs, fat, and calories are not created equal. If you time your food and workouts, you can maximize brain growth while shrinking your waistline.

At first, this diet may be a bit harder to understand than all-or-nothing programs that place strict numbers on the macronutrients of carbohydrates, fat, and protein you consume. You see, the abundance of micronutrients found in vegetables and fruit help you manufacture and sustain healthy levels of serotonin and dopamine, and that allows you to break free from the addiction to sugar and bad fats. You'll feel better in the long run. When you feel good, you're far less likely to crave brain-shrinking foods. Have you ever found that to be true? I know I have.

It's pretty simple. This diet focuses on *adding* the types of foods that the study proving the existence of sugar brain had lots of: high omega-3 sources of fat and protein, vegetables, and whole fruit. It's also flexible. With a few tweaks, vegans can follow it. It's already chock-full of produce. You can follow this eating pattern whether you're vegan, pescatarian, gluten-free, or following a points-based program. Some of the success stories you'll read are from people who followed the Kediterranean-based Sugar Brain Fix and how it helped them to break through a plateau. You'll read success stories from people who were already adhering to points-based diets and added the Sugar Brain Fix to lose even *more* weight. With just a few simple tweaks in 28 days, they lost more fat *and* gained muscle mass.

The Sugar Brain Fix program helped me change my relationship status with sugar and bad fats. We're no longer "in a relationship." The addiction is gone, and the staples of the standard American diet have become once-in-a-while treats. I know that you, too, can put an end to sugar brain. With a bigger brain and a smaller waistline, you'll look, think, and feel better. Before you know it, it will be time to update your relationship status. You'll finally figure out how you and sugar can be "just friends."

How This Book Is Set Up

In Part I, I'll do a deep dive into how sugar affects your brain chemistry, ultimately shrinking your brain and expanding your waistline. You'll learn all about sugar brain: where it comes from and what it feels like. You'll also get a primer on food addiction, willpower, and the gradual detox that makes this program so effective.

In Part II, I'll uncover the relationship between your emotions and your levels of the brain chemicals serotonin or dopamine, or both. You'll take quizzes to help you identify where you're deficient and discover how to manufacture steady levels of these neurotransmitters with a combination of amino acids, vitamins, and minerals—which stops cravings for brain-shrinking foods. You'll also learn about intermittent fasting and mantras, and how these techniques will support you in the program.

In Part III, I'll address special situations and behaviors that can lead to or fuel sugar brain: obsessive eating, emotional eating, and binge eating. Read this section if you identify with any of these conditions or think they might be contributing to your relationship with food and your sugar brain.

In Part IV, we'll heal your sugar brain with the Sugar Brain Fix program. The gradual detox plan I provide will teach you how to fill your plate with foods and activities that grow your brain. You'll supercharge BDNF growth hormone and shred fat with intermittent fasting and fasted workouts. We'll keep your serotonin and dopamine levels steady and grow your brain as you slim your waistline. The power of self-hypnosis, cognitive behavioral therapy, and delicious Sugar Brain Fix–approved recipes will help keep you on track.

Exceptions

There are several conditions that the Sugar Brain Fix program is not intended to address, or only with permission or guidance from your health-care professional. Please see Appendix C on page 313 for more details.

By now, I hope you're intrigued. Perhaps there's part of you that's a bit nervous—especially if you've never tried intermittent fasting or, like I did, you really love your soda. Not to worry. The way the program is set up gradually introduces changes into your life. And if you're like the other people who completed the 28-day Sugar Brain Fix, you'll say it was a lot easier than you expected.

At this point, the most important thing is your motivation for making these changes. When you connect with your *why*, the *what* you need to do becomes exponentially easier. Day by day, you'll start to notice improvements—in the way you think, feel, and look. You'll start to see that happy, healthy version of yourself that, in the long run, is far more rewarding than sugar, wouldn't you agree?

Part I

UNDERSTANDING SUGAR BRAIN

Chapter 1

THE EVOLUTION OF SUGAR BRAIN

To understand sugar brain, it's helpful to go back to the very beginning of your life. For just a moment, imagine yourself as an infant. You ate food made from nature's source of sugar: the fructose, glucose, and sucrose found in fruit. Apples, bananas, and carrots were pureed into a form you could swallow. Along with natural fructose, glucose, and sucrose, you consumed breast milk or formulas with the milk sugar lactose. No matter the form sugar comes in, you're born with an innate preference for sugar. Humans are hard-wired for it on day 1. On the other hand, your preference for fat doesn't develop until you're older.

That innate fondness for sugar is a good thing as an infant. It's nature's way of encouraging you to eat energy-rich foods during this period of rapid growth and development. And even before you learn that a pint of ice cream helps to ease the stress of a bad day, you already inherently possess a brain that will feel less pain with sugar. Research shows that infants who get a little sugar water after a shot cry less. Mary Poppins was right: A spoonful of sugar *does* make the medicine go down.

As an infant, your caretakers decide what and how much you eat. But soon, it becomes apparent that there are some foods you prefer—since you're born with genetically influenced tendencies for tastes. You have unique taste buds that can perceive the sweetness of sugar and pick up on the bitterness of vegetables, and these are set at different levels based on your genes. You also have a unique brain with genetically influenced tendencies that make you predisposed to seek out foods that feel good to your brain's unique neurotransmitter footprint.

Let's look at just one of many examples of genetically influenced tendencies that affect what you eat: your supertaster status. Supertasters have genes that make bitter foods like vegetables taste very pungent, so you're more likely to avoid them and gravitate toward bland foods like carbs. Nontasters have genes that make bitter vegetables taste mild, so eating healthier foods comes easily. That's good, since bitter foods tend to be chock-full of antioxidants and prevent obesity. Your taste buds have a profound effect on your health. Supertasters may have an increased risk of cancer *if* they simply surrender to their initial distaste for vegetables.

It's not all nature, because nurture plays a role as well. If your caretakers expose you to bitter vegetables regularly—despite your initial distaste for them—you'll probably eat them regularly. This example demonstrates an important principle: You're not doomed by your genes. Even if you have genes that predispose you for obesity or for craving certain foods, you can turn those genes *off* by modifying your environment. The number one way to turn off genes or prevent bad genes from ever getting switched *on* is by changing what you eat every day.

As an infant, the foods you consume—milk, fruit juice, and pureed fruits—are all filled with sugars. As they get older, some children develop lactose intolerance. All children develop a taste for fat. Perhaps lactose intolerance is Mother Nature's way of helping you to decrease your consumption of sugars as you reach adulthood. Drinking fruit juice and cow's milk may be okay for kids, but my philosophy is that they're primarily children's drinks. The older you get, the less energy you need. Of course, many adults eat an increasing quantity of food as their metabolism is slowing down with age—a recipe for obesity and a shrunken brain.

A Brief History of Sugar Production in the 18th Century

Now, for a moment, imagine that you were born in the early 1700s, before the era of modern refrigeration. While your mother might not have been spooning liquefied fruit into your mouth, you still had Mother Nature looking out for you. That's because when foods spoil, they'll taste rotten. Before refrigeration and printed due dates on foods, you needed to use this poison-avoidance mechanism. Mother Nature doesn't want you to eat something that will kill you or make you sick.

While Mother Nature doesn't want you eating sugar all the time, she still wants you to eat some sweet foods to optimize your wellness. Whole fruit is nature's dessert. Now that you have teeth, you can bite into that apple; you don't need to drink its juice. There tend to be more vitamins present in fruit as it ripens. So the sweetness that attracts you to whole fruit is there for a purpose. More vitamins mean you won't die from scurvy; vitamins are needed for long-term development and disease prevention.

Since you're imagining yourself in the early 1700s, realize that it was also decades before a few developments that changed brains and waistlines around the world. Around this time, sugar was quite expensive because it was made from sugarcane, which could only grow in tropical climates. Thus, sugar was a hard-to-acquire, once-in-a-while treat. Even if you had cravings, it would have been extremely difficult to consume it all the time.

That all began to change in the mid-1700s, when a German chemist discovered that beetroot contained sugar that was indistinguishable from sugarcane. Sugar could now be extracted from beets as well. This meant it didn't need to be imported from the West Indies. As a result, sugar began to pop up everywhere.

Now, take off your imagination cap and come back to the present. You're an adult and, of course, you don't actually live in the 1700s. You live your life in the processed-food-rich 21st century, where food is available 24/7. You don't even need to get in your car and make it to the drive-through anymore. Just tap on your phone, and someone will bring just about any food you want to your doorstep. Chances are you're not using Uber Eats or Postmates to have organic vegetables delivered. Instead of being a treat, sugar and bad fats are a round-the-clock part of the American diet.

America's Modern-Day Sugar Addiction

Market research provider Euromonitor International surveyed sugar consumption around the world. Of all nationalities surveyed, Americans have the biggest sweet tooth of them all—consuming more sugar per person than any other country. The average American consumes a whopping 126 grams of sugar per day—more than twice the recommended daily intake put forth by the World Health Organization.

And yes, it's *sugar* that is America's primary vice and the one that gets us hooked initially. Surprisingly, Euromonitor found Americans' fat consumption is within healthy guidelines at 65.5 grams per person. While Americans are the number one consumer of sugar, they are not number one in fat consumption. In fact, some countries consume far more fat. For example, the average person in Belgium consumes about 50 percent more fat per day than the average American.

If you had been born in 1700 or prior, your preference for sweet foods kept you healthy since sweet was associated with vitamin-rich. And today's processed foods can sit on shelves for years or be refrigerated, so your taste buds rarely need to aid you in the detection of rotten foods. The irony is that your sense of taste was designed to keep you alive, but most of today's sweet foods will end up killing you if they become your go-to.

While you're harming yourself, you're also harming the planet. In 2019, the EAT-*Lancet* Commission released its findings on healthy diets from sustainable food systems. Thirty-seven scientists from 16 different countries with expertise in both health and environmental sustainability weighed in. You've probably heard how excess consumption of red meat fuels global warming, but most people aren't aware that sugar production is also terrible for the planet.

The commission's recommendation on sugar consumption: It must be cut in half. You see, sugarcane is one of the world's thirstiest crops. About nine gallons of water are required to produce just one teaspoon of sugar. The increasing demand for sugar has fueled deforestation in parts of the world with the most threatened ecosystems, like Brazil. According to the World Wildlife Fund, 12 countries devote at least a quarter of their land for sugarcane production. To meet the projected demand for sugar by 2050, growers will need to allocate 50 percent *more* land to this water-hungry crop.

To help our planet, the EAT-*Lancet* commission also recommended that the consumption of vegetables, fruit, beans, and nuts must double. Good news: The Sugar Brain Fix program is in line with these recommendations. Grow your brain, shrink your waistline, *and* help our planet? That's a win-win-win.

Our modern world sure is a different place than it was just a few hundred years ago. Despite the things that have gotten worse, there are still upsides. Unlike the people in the 1700s, you don't have to worry about dying from smallpox, scarlet fever, or tuberculosis. If you're like most people today, you worry about obesity, diabetes, heart disease, and cancer as soon as you reach adulthood, whereas brain health is often only a concern for people in their 60s, 70s, and beyond. With the recent discovery of sugar brain, brain health is now something that people of all ages should be concerned about. The standard sugar-and-bad-fat-rich American diet isn't just making you gain weight or putting you at risk for a heart attack. It's shrinking your most precious organ: your brain.

The Discovery of Sugar Brain

Sugar brain was discovered in a landmark research study published in 2015 in *BMC Medicine*. This was the first human study that linked a shrunken brain to eating sugar and bad fats, confirming the same phenomenon previously shown in animal studies. This robust study followed hundreds of people over four years. The subjects underwent two MRIs to assess their brains, one at the beginning of the study and a second one four years later.

The researchers examined all the different types of food their subjects ate over the course of several years. Were they eating sugar and sweets? Or vegetables and fruits? Were the fats they consumed good fats or bad fats—more omega-3-rich grilled fish or more omega-6-rich burgers? And how much of each of these foods did they eat? Since they followed their subjects' dietary choices for years, they were able to study long-term effects of food on the brain.

The researchers classified foods into two categories: Western foods and healthy foods. Western foods were those that contained sugar in many different forms and bad fats (like soda, chips, bread, and red and processed meat). Thus, the "sugar" came in the form of added sugar, flour, and grains. Healthy foods were antioxidant-rich vegetables and fruits that don't send blood sugar levels soaring; they also consisted of fat and protein that's high in omega-3s, such as grilled fish.

After the second MRI, researchers could see if a subject's brain had stayed big and beautiful over four years or if it had shrunk. They measured a part of the brain that is particularly prone to volume loss: the hippocampus. Then they correlated brain volume with foods the subjects ate. To make sure a shrinking brain wasn't due to other factors, the researchers accounted for variables like exercise and education.

The five researchers, all affiliated with prestigious universities in Australia, came to a conclusion that made headlines around the world: People who ate lots of sugar and bad fats tended to have shrunken brains—the condition I refer to as sugar brain.

The opposite trend was also found: People who ate nutrient-dense foods that don't send blood sugar soaring, together with omega-3-rich sources of fat and protein, tended to have bigger brains.

Mainstream news outlets picked up the published research, and it radically changed the way I thought about food—and what I ate.

While this study looked at associations, cause-and-effect animal studies have demonstrated the way that introducing sugar damages the brain. One study gave one group of baby rats sugar water while others got plain water. The sugar damaged the brain in profound ways.

Another study fed animals sugar and bad fats and then measured BDNF levels. No surprise: Sugar and bad fats made this brain-growing hormone plummet. The good news: Another cause-and-effect study injected rats with BDNF; the growth hormone helped obese rats who were previously fed a Western diet to lose weight.

It's more proof that while sugar and bad fats shrink your brain and expand your waistline, their effects can be reversed.

Next, we'll take a deeper dive into sugar and bad fats to fully understand them. They're a bit complicated, and this is compounded by the fact that food companies disguise them so that you won't see the words *sugar* or *soybean oil* on their ingredients list. To fix sugar brain, it's important to understand what "sugar" and "bad fats" mean. You'll learn which ones to avoid and what carbs and fats you can use to replace them.

Sugar

The *BMC Medicine* sugar brain study found it wasn't just added white sugar that was linked to a shrunken brain. Flour, potatoes, and grains were brain-shrinking foods as well. Because of the way they spike blood sugar rapidly, all of these foods are essentially sugar at their most basic form. The only carbohydrate sources linked to a bigger brain were vegetables (not including potatoes) and whole fruits.

Because of the way they help grow your brain, no whole fruits are off limits. As I mentioned in the introduction, vegetables are permitted except for all types of potato.

Since corn can be classified as a vegetable or a grain, it falls into many categories. If it's whole corn or popcorn, it's permitted. Corn that's been ground in the form of chips or tortillas is not, since that form of corn has been linked to a shrunken brain. Grains were also linked to a shrunken brain; thus, they are not part of the Sugar Brain Fix program. Grains spike blood sugar and disrupt fat-burning ketosis. That being said, the Sugar Brain Fix program always allows for at least two or more reasonable servings of any food you like by the time you make it to the fourth week of the 28-day program. If you'd like, you can have rice, chips, sugar, or flour—but you'll begin to limit your servings. Eating these foods occasionally won't shrink your brain instantly and, as you'll learn, doesn't set you up for addiction to these foods.

It's also important to recognize all the forms sugar comes in since food companies try and trick consumers by calling sugar by different names. Note that artificial sweeteners are not part of the Sugar Brain Fix because of the way they can affect your brain and blood sugar levels via the gut-brain connection. If you're looking for a sweetener, stevia is permitted on the Sugar Brain Fix program. As for sugar alcohols, a small amount of xylitol is acceptable in things like sugar-free gum. Maltitol can increase blood sugar, so avoid this sugar alcohol.

Philosophically, the Sugar Brain Fix isn't about replacing foods with low- or no-calorie foods; it's about filling your diet with healthy foods like vegetables and whole fruits. So the focus is generally to move away from sugar-free candies or diet foods that use sugar alcohols in an effort to grow your brain and shrink your waistline.

Whenever I say the word *sugar* in this book, here's what I mean:

- Ace-K or acesulfame-K
- Agave nectar/syrup
- Amaranth
- Aspartame
- Barley
- Barley malt
- Beet sugar
- Blackstrap molasses
- Brown rice syrup
- Brown sugar
- Buckwheat
- Bulgur
- Buttered sugar/ buttercream
- Cane juice crystals
- Cane sugar
- Caramel
- Carob syrup
- Castor sugar
- Coconut sugar
- Confectioner's sugar (aka, powdered sugar)
- Corn syrup
- Corn syrup solids
- Crystalline fructose
- Date sugar
- Demerara sugar
- Dextrin
- Dextrose
- Diastatic malt
- Einkorn
- Equal
- Ethyl maltol
- Evaporated cane juice
- Farro
- Florida crystals
- Flour (all except almond, coconut, teff, and tigernut)
- Fructose
- Fruit juice
- Fruit juice concentrate
- Galactose
- Golden sugar
- Golden syrup
- Glucose
- Glucose syrup solids
- Grape sugar
- Grains
- High-fructose corn syrup (HFCS)
- Honey
- Icing sugar
- Invert sugar
- Kamut
- Kaniwa
- Lactose
- Malt syrup
- Maltodextrin
- Maltose
- Maple syrup
- Millet
- Molasses
- Muscovado sugar
- Oats
- Panela sugar
- Quinoa
- Raw sugar
- Rice (all)
- Rice syrup

- Refiners syrup
- Saccharin
- Sorghum syrup
- Spelt
- Splenda
- Sucralose
- Sucrose
- Sugar (granulated or table)
- Sucanat
- Sunett
- Sweet One
- Sweet'N Low
- Turbinado sugar
- Treacle
- Wheat
- Yellow sugar

Bad Fats

Like sugar, fats are complex. Fats come in different forms: trans, saturated, polyunsaturated, and monounsaturated. The fat in the Sugar Brain Fix diet comes mostly from antioxidant-rich olive oil, which is almost all good monounsaturated fat. It replaces the most prevalent oils in the Western diet, including soybean oil, which has high levels of bad fats: saturated fat and polyunsaturated fat. This one simple swap goes a long way in replacing bad fats with good ones. Due to the type of fat they contain, cold- or expeller-pressed canola, walnut, avocado, macadamia nut, and Malaysian palm fruit oils are also permitted.

The Western diet is filled with trans fats and low-quality saturated fat in the form of conventionally raised animal products and processed foods. The Sugar Brain Fix Kediterranean diet does include small amounts of saturated fat, but these fats differ from those found in the Western diet. Small amounts of virgin coconut oil, grass-fed butter, grass-fed ghee, and MCT oil are permitted, because these fats are higher in medium-chain triglycerides, whereas the saturated fat in the Western diet is filled with long-chain triglycerides. Unlike long-chain triglycerides, medium-chain triglycerides can help you lose weight and *lower* cholesterol. Additionally, the Sugar Brain Fix diet encourages small amounts of healthy saturated fats to paradoxically *decrease* your overall intake of saturated fats. For many people, a teaspoon or two of good fats actually helps them to decrease cravings and consumption of a day's worth of bad fats.

That being said, the Sugar Brain Fix diet tends to be much lower in saturated fats than traditional keto. If you do put a good fat in your morning coffee, use just a teaspoon or two. While fat doesn't spike blood sugar and insulin as much as carbohydrates, too much fat can interfere with mild ketosis during intermittent fasting—so limit this fat to a very small amount.

The other difference in fat sources is the ratio of anti-inflammatory omega-3s to pro-inflammatory omega-6s. The best source of usable omega-3 in your diet is fish. No surprise: Grilled fish was the one protein/fat source linked to a bigger brain in the *BMC Medicine* sugar brain study. As part of your 28-day program, you'll eat one omega-3-rich food daily. Omega-6-rich food was linked to a shrunken brain in the sugar brain study. Thus, you'll start decreasing the amount of conventionally raised meat, dairy, and eggs in your diet, since they have higher levels of omega-6s and lower omega-3s than those labeled grass-fed, organic, pastured, or free-range. You'll also limit all processed meats since they were also linked to a shrunken brain. This means *all* types of processed meat, including all lunch meats.

To recap, you'll want to avoid the following *bad fats*:

- Fried foods
- High-omega-6 foods (e.g., all conventionally raised animal products, including dairy and eggs)
- Lunch meat, including all cold cuts and deli meats (e.g., turkey, ham, etc.)
- Margarine
- Processed meat
- Red meat—except those with higher levels of omega-3s like grass-fed, organic varieties
- Saturated fat (except a tablespoon of virgin coconut oil or high-omega-3 saturated fat in organic, grass-fed, free-range animal products)
- Trans fats

What Does Sugar Brain *Feel* Like?

The first piece of the sugar brain puzzle is answering this question: Why would people be compelled to keep eating foods that shrink their brains? Now that we know this, why can't we just simply stop? The answer: The immediate serotonin and dopamine release of sugar and bad fats makes you want to keep eating them. You become *addicted* to foods that shrink your brain.

The addictive pull of sugar and bad fats can be seen in brain scans as they light up your brain's reward centers. One recent study conducted by researchers in Oregon who specialize in eating pathology compared the way sugar and fat affect the brain. Subjects consumed two different milk shakes: a high-fat one and one with lots of sugar. As they were doing so, their brains were scanned. Sugar was even more effective than fat at lighting up the brain's rewards centers. No wonder food companies layer sugar into almost everything, including products that already contain bad fats. Many foods most people think of as fat—like most store-bought dressings—actually contain sugar.

The second piece of the puzzle is knowing how it *feels* when you have sugar brain. After all, sugar brain isn't technically a diagnosis recognized by your health insurance company! But if you eat sugar and bad fats regularly, this shrinks your hippocampus, so you're more likely to be diagnosed with other conditions your health insurance company *does* recognize: depression, mild cognitive impairment, or impulse-control disorders.

The shrunken hippocampus that occurs when you have sugar brain has been linked to three different emotions or patterns of behavior to watch out for. If you have mild sugar brain, you'll probably notice one or two of these feelings. If you've been shrinking your brain for decades like I did, you may notice all of them.

First, sugar brain may make you feel *blue,* since a shrunken hippocampus can negatively affect your ability to regulate your mood. If this goes on for years, sugar brain may even lead to depression—since the foods that shrink your brain also cause inflammation throughout the brain and body. In recent years, science has shown that inflammation can trigger depression in many individuals. In fact, depression itself has been referred to as an inflammatory disease.

Second, sugar brain may make you feel *impulsive*, since having a shrunken hippocampus has been linked to impulsivity. You see that food and know you shouldn't have it. But it just feels so hard to resist. With an impulsive shrunken brain, you don't resist.

Third, sugar brain can make you feel *stuck*. A shrunken hippocampus can change your emotional responses and affect decision-making skills. This affects your everyday behavior as you become inflexible and less able to change the way you think and act, so the bad decisions continue. This is because your hippocampus isn't just about memory; it talks to the emotional amygdala as it encodes and stores emotionally charged memories. When you encounter something that makes you feel positive or negative emotions in the future, the hippocampus affects the way the amygdala will respond.

In Part II, we'll delve more into emotional states linked to sugar brain and how we can stop craving sugar once and for all.

Sugar, Memory, and the Downward Spiral of Addiction

Let's look at an example of how sugar brain may affect you in your everyday life, and how three parts of your brain get involved: the hypothalamus, the hippocampus, and the amygdala. Think about all the times you've had birthday cake in your life. You're enjoying that sweet, moist cake topped with buttercream icing, and you're having fun as you celebrate. Let's say it's the first time you've ever eaten cake, at your first birthday party. Even without a memory of this food or an event, serotonin and dopamine are released instantly. Pleasure pathways in the brain send signals to the hypothalamus, which is responsible for regulating food intake. When you're full, a message is sent to the hypothalamus to stop eating. Naturally, this becomes harder when the pleasure pathways override signs for physical hunger.

SEROTONIN AND DOPAMINE → PLEASURE
PATHWAYS → HYPOTHALAMUS (PHYSICAL HUNGER)

When all of this is happening, your hippocampus is storing memories. Since you're feeling something emotional when this happens, your hippocampus talks to your amygdala. Sugar and bad fats have sent serotonin and dopamine soaring, so you already feel really good. Hopefully, you're also having a great time with friends. Now a positive life experience is getting linked to food.

Of course, negative experiences can get paired and stored, too. Let's say you're going through a breakup and turn to a pint of ice cream to console you and make you feel better in the short term. Now memory and emotion add to the initial chemical response of dopamine and serotonin that get sent to the hypothalamus, making eating brain-shrinking foods more likely when you're emotional.

HIPPOCAMPUS (MEMORY) ⟷ AMYGDALA (EMOTION)

When a hippocampus is functioning properly, it's easier to resist triggers. But a shrunken hippocampus makes it harder since you're more likely to feel blue, stuck, or impulsive.

A healthy hippocampus will store memories of every meal, which helps you to not eat as much at your next meal. One study inserted a special gene into the hippocampus of rats that allowed researchers to turn off this part of the brain by shining a certain type of light on them. Turning off the hippocampus with a light after a meal had a profound effect on food consumption. Without a functioning hippocampus, the rats ate their next meal sooner and consumed double the amount of food during that meal compared to when that special light was turned off and the hippocampus was functioning.

So when your hippocampus is healthy, it will store a memory of every meal, helping you to eat less often and smaller portions. You're also more likely to feel happy and have good impulse control. When this is all true, you can easily listen to the signs of physical hunger you're receiving from the hypothalamus. But with a shrunken hippocampus, you don't listen to these signals—because of the impaired memory, alluring emotionally charged memories, and an impaired ability to change your behavior.

Every time you go to another birthday party, have another bad day, see a piece of cake or a pint of ice cream, the hippocampus is retrieving previous memories that have been stored, changing the way the emotional amygdala responds. You remember how all that sugar and bad fat made you feel better— at least for the short term. A craving is born. You don't *need* the food, but you *want* it. You go for a second piece. And the more you do, the more the hippocampus shrinks. Do that 100 times, and you've created a pathway of deeply ingrained behavior. A habit. An addiction.

Let's look at this downward spiral. The more you eat sugars and bad fats, the more you become addicted to them. The more addicted to them you become, the more you eat them. The more you eat them, the more you shrink your hippocampus. The more you shrink your hippocampus, the more you feel blue, stuck, impulsive, and foggy. The more you feel this way, the more you eat sugar and bad fats. And so on.

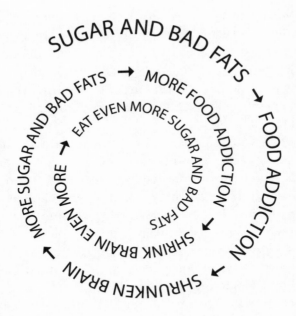

To fully understand how sugar brain develops, we first have to fully understand food addiction, since that's how this chain reaction's fuse gets lit. The initial release of serotonin and dopamine was the first domino, and then other dominos topple as other parts of the brain are affected. By understanding the chemical reaction of food, you'll understand how and why your sugar brain developed.

As you'll learn in this book, some people's neurochemistry makes them particularly prone to the lure of either sugar *or* fat as the primary culprit. The quizzes I've provided in Part II will help you to determine your own personal neurochemistry, which will help you to understand why you're so drawn to sugar, bad fats, or both. Both can shrink your brain as the addictive lure makes you unable to stop.

Next we'll take a look at the role of willpower in the brain. By understanding how food can hijack your self-control, you'll be better equipped to take the power back.

Chapter 2

WILLPOWER IS NOT THE PROBLEM

*I think you can properly regard food addiction as
somewhat similar to drug addiction. If you can help
people to at least reduce their craving levels, you'll
contribute a lot to solving the obesity epidemic.*

— TUNG FONG, DIRECTOR OF METABOLIC DISEASES RESEARCH AT
DRUGMAKER MERCK & CO., IN THE *CHICAGO TRIBUNE,* 2005

My patient Rosemary sat across from me, gripping the arm-rests of her chair and speaking quickly and softly, almost in a whisper. It was as though by muffling her words she could keep them from being true. Rosemary had been reluctant to talk about her compulsive eating in previous sessions. Today, Rosemary was finally ready to talk about her frequent bouts of secret eating. Like so many of us, she was totally hooked on sugar.

"I'm just so ashamed," she kept saying as she detailed her struggles to control her weight. "I don't know how I ever let it get this bad." First, she explained, she had been satisfied with an occasional candy bar at work, a sugar rush that helped her get through the most stressful "deadline days" at the online magazine where she reviewed computer software. Then she'd started having dessert at lunch—a brownie, a piece of cake, a frosted muffin. Somehow her lunchtime treat had expanded into a dinnertime ritual, then a breakfast Danish, then a second candy bar. Now, Rosemary explained, she was essentially eating sugar all day long, a fact that embarrassed her so greatly that she could barely look at me as she spoke.

"So you think this is all your fault," I said carefully when she fell into a long silence, her hands still gripping the armrests.

"Whose fault is it? Nobody put a gun to my head." She forced herself to meet my eyes.

I often encounter a sense of shame like Rosemary's, whether my patients are struggling with food addictions or substance abuse. In fact, the feelings underneath both conditions are strikingly similar. Most of us like to feel powerful and in control. Acknowledging an addiction makes us feel weak and helpless. It's as though our brain chemistry, and not us, was suddenly in charge of our destiny. Even if we know we're shrinking our brains, we feel powerless to do anything about it. Rosemary felt blue, stuck, and impulsive—all clues that she, indeed, had sugar brain.

When my patients can accept that *willpower is not the problem,* they often feel liberated and relieved. When Rosemary understood the brain chemistry of food addiction that leads to sugar brain, she began to view herself with more compassion.

"Maybe I'm being too hard on myself," she told me at one session. "I thought I could just stop eating sweets—and then I didn't understand why I *wasn't* stopping. But you're telling me that I was actually developing a physical addiction to sugar. Like an addict, I needed more and more and more—and if I tried to cut back, I felt so awful I could hardly stand it."

She took a deep breath. "So it wasn't just willpower," she said, repeating the words I had once said to her. "I was actually going through withdrawal."

In fact, Rosemary had been going through a rapid, almost violent detox, certain to produce unpleasant and often painful symptoms that were virtually guaranteed to sabotage her efforts to give up brain-shrinking foods. Later in this book, I'll show you how to go through *gradual* detox, so that your Sugar Brain Fix is painless and even pleasurable.

First, though, let's find out what Rosemary learned. Let's understand exactly what it means to be addicted to food that shrinks our brains.

Scientific Proof: Food Addiction Exists!

In March 2010, the Scripps Research Institute released a groundbreaking study. Rats who were fed sugar-and-bad-fat-filled diets of bacon, sausage, chocolate, and cheesecake developed full-blown *food addictions*: actual neurochemical dependencies as powerful as those caused by cocaine.

In the study, rats were given different kinds of access to these brain-shrinking foods. Some were limited to only an hour of human treats a day, while others were allowed to eat bacon and chocolate virtually around the clock. While the rats with limited access ate moderately and were able to maintain their weight, the rats with more access quickly became obese—and obsessed.

It was astonishing how far those food-addicted rats would go to maintain their habit. When researchers withheld the junk food and tried to put the rats back on a healthy diet, the obese rats refused to eat, almost to the point of starvation. The rats would even choose to endure painful shocks to get the junk food. Their desperation to stuff themselves with foods made from sugar and bad fats—and their willingness to endure pain in its service—was strikingly similar to those of rats in different studies who had become addicted to other substances that also shrink the brain: cocaine and heroin.

Using special electrodes to monitor the rats' responses, researchers discovered that foods with sugar and bad fats had changed the animals' brain chemistry—in virtually identical ways to cocaine or heroin. Both excessive junk food and other types of drugs overload the brain's pleasure centers. Like Rosemary, the rats needed ever-larger quantities of sweet, fatty food to get the same "high." The more often you get high, the more the brain shrinks.

We tend to think that food's comfort is an emotional issue and blame ourselves for being childlike or weak. But rats don't have psychological issues, and yet they were behaving exactly like food-obsessed humans. Because of the way the food had altered their brain chemistry, these overweight and food-addicted rats *physically* needed more and more junk food to experience pleasure—or just to feel normal. Unlimited access to these foods had turned them into addicts.

Now here's the even scarier part: After cocaine-addicted rats stopped taking the drug, it took only two days for their brain chemistry to return to normal. For the food-addicted rats in the food study, though, their brain chemistry took *two weeks* to return to normal. In some ways, food habits affected the brain *more* than drugs. Unlike triggers for drugs, which can be minimized with planning, triggers for food are everywhere. You don't need drugs to stay alive, but you do need food.

The Scripps study shows that we can no longer view unhealthy eating as a matter of willpower. After all, rats don't have emotional issues, childhood histories, or deep-seated associations between food and love. They know only what their brain chemistry tells them. And the obese rats were hearing the message loud and clear: *Go for the bacon and cheesecake.* This new research suggests that drug addiction and food addiction are products of the same neurobiology. That means that sugar and bad fats can be as addictive as crack. Most people eat brain-shrinking foods more frequently than most drug addicts get high, because they do it every few hours, every single day.

The Scripps study also showed that these foods don't *have* to take over our lives, *if* we enjoy them in limited amounts. You can learn to be "just friends" with sugar and bad fats. That group of rats that was allowed to eat only bacon-and cheesecake-type foods for one hour each day enjoyed their treats, but they did not become addicted. Nor did they gain much weight. They had access to seductive "pitfall" foods—but that access was *limited*. As a result, they never became addicted, and their weights remained normal. In fact, their weight was quite similar to a group of rats who were *never* given "pitfall" foods and who were fed only rat chow. But the rats who had access to high-sugar, bad-fat-filled foods around the clock experienced immediate weight gain. The rats became obese quickly, and their weight spiraled out of control.

Dopamine: The Body's Energizer

Let's take a closer look at what was going on in the addicted rats' brains. All of us—rats and humans alike—respond to the brain chemical dopamine, an energizing, vitalizing substance that our brains produce in response to pleasure and excitement. When you ride a roller coaster, gamble for high stakes, or go on a thrilling romantic date, your dopamine levels rise. When you feel listless and bored, your dopamine levels have fallen.

Dopamine is responsible for the rush you feel when you first fall in love. It's also one of the brain chemicals that is stimulated by cocaine. That's why people who use the drug feel jazzed up, wide awake, and filled with short-lived pleasure. When you think about how good dopamine makes us feel, whether from healthy sources or unhealthy ones, it's hard not to want to be flooded with it all the time.

But here's the problem: The body was not designed for a 24-hour high, whether from romance, cocaine, or anything else. Sooner or later, what goes up must come down. And too great or too intense a thrill inevitably produces a crash.

If you've just gotten back from your first trip to Paris, for example, maybe you feel a little let down your first day back at work. Paperwork seems mundane. Your favorite TV show seems dull. All you want is to get back to the exciting, dopamine-releasing newness that made your heart sing.

Likewise, coming down from a cocaine high is disappointing at best, painful at worst. You feel tired, listless, and burnt out. You usually feel lower than before you did the cocaine in the first place.

So what causes that crash? In most cases, your body has used up your dopamine stores too quickly. After a few hours of excitement, your body just can't keep up. Your dopamine stores temporarily run out, and you have even less than you usually do. You feel flat, listless, exhausted, and let down. Time for a rest, so the body can make more dopamine.

Ideally, we'll get nice, level doses of dopamine that keep us "up" and happy but that aren't so intense and abrupt that they're followed by a crash. That's what happens normally and will keep your brain big and beautiful. But what if, like the rats in the study, you are continually pumping up your dopamine levels with regular infusions of "exciting" foods made from bad fats? Then, like the rats, you may come to depend on those foods, not for excitement but just to feel normal. Over time, this ends up shrinking your brain.

Keeping Your Brain in Balance

Our brains are amazing chemical systems. They are designed to keep a nice, steady balance with just the right chemical levels to keep us happy and allow us to function. We have in our brains pretty much all the chemicals we need to recover from pain, rise to a challenge, enjoy a thrill, or just feel good.

When a biochemical reaction modifies your brain chemistry, however, all sorts of problems occur. Suppose you eat a bacon cheeseburger or a nice big bag of chips. You've just cued your brain to release more dopamine, which is why you get that short-lived rush of pleasure.

Indulging might be fine if you did it only occasionally. But if you overdo the bad-fat foods, your brain chemistry begins to change. The neurons that release, receive, and keep dopamine moving through your brain first become overloaded, then damaged. They can't carry dopamine as efficiently as they once did. As a result, you need greater and greater quantities of dopamine to compensate for these overworked neurons.

Meanwhile, by giving yourself a big, extra jolt of those chemicals, you've confused your brain. Soon, instead of producing its own dopamine slowly and steadily, it "waits" for that big chemical jolt and then produces a flood of dopamine in response. Gradually, your brain begins to depend on that jolt from the outside. Instead of sticking to its own internal, stable rhythm, it responds to those hefty doses of bad fats.

Now that your dopamine neurons are damaged, you need even more dopamine than you did before to feel normal. That outside jolt—the extra fat in your cheeseburger—has to get bigger and bigger and bigger. Where once a single cheeseburger could give you that dopamine rush, now you need two cheeseburgers and a double order of fries. Over time, this shrinks your brain as it expands your waistline. The more you shrink your brain, the harder it is to say no to foods that give you a dopamine rush—so bring on yet another cheeseburger.

> BAD FATS → EXCESS DOPAMINE → OVERWORKED NEURONS → NEED MORE DOPAMINE TO FEEL NORMAL → EAT *MORE* BAD FATS → DAMAGED NEURONS → NEED MORE DOPAMINE TO FEEL NORMAL → EAT *MORE* BAD FATS → MORE FLOODING → MORE DAMAGE → NEED EVEN *MORE* DOPAMINE → SHRINK THE BRAIN → EAT EVEN *MORE* BAD FATS . . .

Just as the bingeing rats found out, unrestricted access to unhealthy foods creates a vicious cycle. The more you eat, the more you want. Your brain chemistry starts to need ever-higher amounts of the outside substance just to function at all as you become less able to manage your moods.

So what happens when you eat a fat, juicy cheeseburger every day for six months and then suddenly switch to a nice bed of greens with chickpeas, organic chicken, and olive oil? Your brain chemistry is seriously disrupted. Since the cheeseburgers had been helping to flood your system with dopamine, your brain now needs more fat than the average, healthy brain just to get a normal dopamine response. So when that salad *doesn't* generate lots of dopamine, your brain is at a loss. It needs dopamine but it doesn't have any, and the only way it knows how to get more is to be supplied, once again, with those bad fats. It's harder to change your ways, because having a shrunken brain makes you feel blue, stuck, impulsive, and foggy.

That's where your cravings begin. That salad might have tasted delicious, but if it doesn't give you huge quantities of bad fats, it leaves you feeling listless, let down, and depressed. As we'll see in Chapter 3, you start to have actual withdrawal symptoms, just like a cocaine addict, including sleep disorders, memory problems, difficulty concentrating, and a general feeling of intense discomfort.

Sooner or later, your brain will realize that it has to start making its own dopamine, and slowly production starts again. But remember how long it took the rats in that study to resume eating normally? Two whole weeks. That's how long it takes your brain to kick back into gear.

Serotonin: Feeling Calm, Peaceful, and Positive

The Scripps study wasn't the only one to deal with food addictions. In 2008, another study confirmed that rats can become addicted to sugar. This study showed rats manifesting responses remarkably similar to those of humans: cravings for the sweet stuff, anxiety-based withdrawal, and then a manic, *increased* desire to binge on sugar.

This time, though, the rats were craving not dopamine but serotonin. Serotonin is the feel-good substance that helps us feel calm, at peace, optimistic, and positive about ourselves. People with low serotonin levels feel anxious and pessimistic and suffer from low self-esteem. Low serotonin levels have been implicated in sleep problems and migraines, as well as in depression and mood disorders such as chronic anxiety and obsessive-compulsive disorder. Interestingly, heroin addicts often report powerful sugar cravings as they try to detox from their addictive substance, suggesting a strong connection between sugar and the pleasure centers that heroin stimulates.

Also interesting is the fact that when people diagnosed with depression are given meds to boost their serotonin levels, they not only cheer up but also begin to feel more optimistic about the future and express higher levels of confidence and self-esteem. Just that simple switch in brain chemistry helps them go from "I'll never find a job; who would want to hire me?" to "You know, there was an ad in the paper that looked interesting—I think I'll check it out." Or perhaps "I'm so fat and ugly, no one will want me" turns into "Actually, I'm a terrific person with a lot of great friends, and I feel hopeful that someday I'll meet a great partner, too." Serotonin is integrally bound up in our view of the world, our predictions for the future, and our feelings about ourselves.

So how do you boost your serotonin levels? Sugar will boost them—temporarily. This includes foods made from flour, including pasta, crackers, grains, bread, and rice. And, as with the unhealthy dopamine boosters we just looked at, the sugar high is inevitably followed by a sugar crash. After the sugar wears off, you feel *worse* than you did before. You have to keep eating more and more sugar just to get the same high—and eventually, just to feel normal. You're compelled to keep doing something that is shrinking your brain as it expands your waistline. On the other hand, healthy foods with the right mix of amino acids, vitamins, and minerals help you to sustain serotonin without the crash.

Later in this book, I'll show you ways that you can naturally change the self-critical, negative thought patterns that might be holding you back into self-loving, positive messages. In Part IV, we'll use self-hypnosis to plant affirmations about your worth deep into your subconscious brain, and cognitive behavior therapy to heal and grow your brain. It's striking that our brain chemistry has so much to do with whether we are able to generate these messages for ourselves or even hear and believe them from others. If your serotonin stores are low, you can hear all the compliments or good advice in the world, and you may very well feel hopeless or anxious anyway. Boosting your serotonin levels is often crucial to any other kind of psychological progress.

Most of us are aware that sweets and starches feel comforting, but we've probably come to believe that's an emotional reaction. Maybe so, but its roots are definitely physical. In a brain-scan study conducted in 2004, scientists found that just the sight and thought of ice cream stimulated the same brain pleasure centers in healthy people as pictures of crack pipes did for drug addicts. Both eating food and thinking about it are deeply biological experiences as well as profoundly emotional ones. If we *feel* addicted to food, it's because we *are*. Even if we know that these foods are shrinking our brains, we can't stop.

Diets Don't Work—Tackling the Way Food Affects Your Brain Does

People aren't stupid. Most of us know that when we feel blue, stressed, or out of control, eating won't solve the problem. That's why we feel so bad about not sticking to a healthy diet. "I *know* this isn't good for me," we tell ourselves. "But I can't control myself! What's *wrong* with me? Why am I so weak?"

Well, now you know that you aren't weak at all—you're simply responding to your own brain chemistry. Overconsumption of sugar and bad fats has taught your body to stop making its own dopamine or serotonin, while tolerance has caused you to need ever-greater quantities of those tempting foods just to feel normal. Take away the addictive foods too suddenly and, like a cocaine addict, you'll go into withdrawal. Unlike someone who has used cocaine, though, your withdrawal symptoms won't last two days. They'll go on for *two weeks*. The more your brain shrinks, the harder it is to change.

In many ways, the way your brain and body adapt is part of the problem. Tolerance is your brain's mechanism to protect itself.

If you eat too much sugar and bad fats, your brain says, "Whoa! If I keep releasing this much serotonin and dopamine, we're going to have a problem." Through another mechanism of self-preservation, the body's basal metabolic rate will decrease with fixed, daily caloric restriction—so you burn less energy. No wonder traditional diets often fail. The Sugar Brain Fix diet is a way around these problems. By substituting serotonin and dopamine boosters for addictive sugar and bad fats, you can still get a steady supply of feel-good neurotransmitters. If you vary eating patterns with intermittent fasting, your body won't ever have a chance to adjust and slow your metabolism.

In Chapters 12 and 13, I'll show you exactly how you can prevent withdrawal symptoms and maintain your brain chemicals with replacement foods and activities—so that you never have to feel deprived or uncomfortable while you are changing your diet and growing your brain. But I hope now you're beginning to see why all your other diets haven't worked so well. All those other diets relied on willpower. "If only I could be disciplined," we tell ourselves. "If only I could stop being so lazy and so greedy!" So we Atkins, calorie- or carb-count, and Blood Type Diet our way to insanity. Do you know anyone who has sustained a no-carb or keto diet for years? I don't. Severely restrictive diets are usually pretty unrealistic in the long term.

Even after you've had some success on a particular diet—even if that diet offers you healthy choices and a sustainable number of calories—you probably found yourself slipping after a few months. Why?

Again, it's not that you lack willpower. It's that you never focused on feeding and growing your brain. Without the physical and emotional support you need, your brain is starving for the serotonin you got from sugar and desperate for the dopamine in your bad-fat-rich snacks.

If your life is stressful or if you feel chronically anxious and unsafe, your serotonin levels probably have been low for a while, making you all the more vulnerable to the power of sugar. Likewise, if your life feels boring and restricted, if you chronically feel blue and lethargic, your dopamine levels have likely dropped even before you started worrying about your weight.

How the Sugar Brain Fix Program Will Help

I'm going to tell you something that might seem a little strange at first: Keep eating all the brain-shrinking foods you're now eating. Do you eat candy bars at every meal? Great! You can continue eating candy bars for the first two weeks of the Sugar Brain Fix program.

My approach to fixing your sugar brain is based on gradual detox, in which you begin by adding healthy foods that will boost your serotonin and dopamine levels before you ever cut back on *anything*. It's vital that we come from a psychological place of plenty. We need to start out knowing that there is nothing we cannot have if we really want it.

Here's how forcing ourselves to diet cold turkey creates a weight-*gain* cycle:

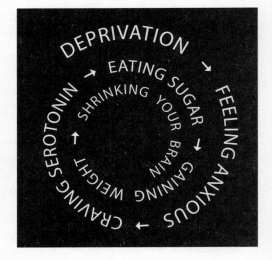

If I'm treating a patient who wants to quit smoking, I tell them they should continue to smoke for a month after making the decision to quit. I realize that might sound odd, but I'll explain. A habit is fully formed in 28 days. So we spend 28 days *adding* to their life before we take the smoking away. We add activities such as running, yoga, and improving relationships. We start to explore the replacement options we'll have on hand once the smoking stops, like patches or the medication Zyban, which is yet another way to increase dopamine levels to counteract the effects of nicotine withdrawal. Add some self-hypnosis to these cognitive behavioral techniques, and you've got a recipe for lasting success.

Can you see what we've used that month to do? The nicotine addict has now formed new habits that boost the same neuro-chemicals he or she has gotten from smoking. After raising these levels, then—and only then—should we remove the nicotine from their system. At that point, the person will hardly notice the loss, because they'll be getting so much dopamine from so many other sources.

The same principle applies to food, especially sugar. Even when you fit someone with a gastric band, if you don't address their brain, they'll continue to feel miserable and deprived. They'll still crave the foods that made them feel good—that did, actually, generate the brain chemicals that we all need to feel good—and then, as happens to some 40 percent of the people who have this procedure, they aren't able to stick to the recommended changes in diet just months after the procedure. We all have to feed our brains with the right foods and activities or we'll never be able to give up the addiction.

In the Sugar Brain Fix program, we address your brain chemistry. You'll learn how to naturally boost your serotonin and dopamine levels, creating the feelings of peace, calm, excitement, and pleasure that you used to get mainly from food. When your brain chemistry is balanced, you'll be interested in food for pleasure, yes, but you won't be dependent on it. It will finally return to its rightful place in your life, and your waistline and brain will show it.

Finding Freedom from Sugar

I remember the first time I helped free someone from a food addiction. My patient Michelle—a longtime sugar addict—and I had been working for weeks on creating new, healthy habits to drive out the old, addictive behaviors. For a while, as in any process of recovery, it was tough going. Michelle was a fighter, no question about that. Although she was not yet 30, she had already been through a lot: an intense battle with stomach cancer, a subtly abusive boyfriend, and a long string of dead-end jobs.

Now she was finally working in an office where her boss and colleagues appreciated her, and she was looking at programs for going back to school. For the first time in years she wasn't dating, which she viewed as her chance to come into her own and discover who she was. She had recently joined a softball team, started cooking more often, and had just about reached her ideal weight.

One day she burst into my office, grinning from ear to ear. "You'll never guess," she began, before I even had a chance to ask her how she was. "I was walking by my favorite bakery, and I was thinking so hard about this new project at work, and this idea I had for what they could do, and the way I was going to convince them to put me in charge, that I walked right past it! I've never done that before! I didn't even notice. I even told myself that I could go back, if I wanted to, and get myself a doughnut—I've been pretty on target lately, and it was time for a treat. But you know what? I just didn't feel like it. Dr. Mike, I can't believe it! I never thought I just wouldn't feel like eating sugar!" Michelle was describing freedom from addiction, and for her it was a beautiful feeling.

Are you wondering whether that could ever be you? Don't worry, I promise you that it can. If you're eager to get started, turn to page 235 and begin your 28-day Sugar Brain Fix. But I'd love for you to read through the next few chapters, because the more fully you understand what is going on in your brain and body, the better choices you'll be able to make and the more motivated you'll be to carry them out.

Chapter 3

HOW FOOD ADDICTION FUELS SUGAR BRAIN— AND VICE VERSA

My patient Sondra was a tall, striking woman whose blond hair fell to her shoulders in long, flowing waves. She worked out regularly at her gym, taking a thrice-weekly spin class and lifting weights with a personal trainer. Every morning she carefully prepared a healthy breakfast of egg whites and half a grapefruit, and every afternoon she ate the salad with grilled chicken that she had brought to work from home.

Yet Sondra was at least 40 pounds overweight, and she had gained 15 of those pounds in the past three months.

"I was doing okay there for a while," she told me, trying to smile through what was obviously a difficult conversation. "I was on a new diet—not Atkins, that was last year; and I did South Beach the year before; and the Zone the year before that! But this one was new, and it was working really great! For a while . . . And then . . ."

Her voice trailed off. "What happened?" I finally asked.

She shook her head. "What always happens," she said flatly. "The new diet works great, I lose a bunch of weight, then something messes me up—my boyfriend or my mom or something at work or—I don't even know what. But all of a sudden, I just can't stick to the new diet anymore, no matter how hard I try, and then bam! I start eating chocolate and bacon and muffins and cookies—I really love those black-and-white cookies, you know, with the frosting?—and then I gain back all the weight I lost plus another 5 or 10 pounds on top. Then I start a new diet, lose some of the weight, and feel really great—until I screw everything up again."

Sondra was struggling with a very common aspect of food addiction: yo-yo weight gain. Through sheer determination she would force herself to follow a strict diet, suffering through the pain of withdrawal from foods rich in sugars and bad fats until her addiction was seemingly broken. She'd go on to eat a healthy diet, lose some weight, and feel terrific.

Then a crisis would hit—nothing major, necessarily, but the normal wear and tear of daily life. Sometimes she'd have a fight with her boyfriend. Other times her mother would make a new demand, or her boss would set a tough deadline, or she'd stress about her growing credit card debt. The anxiety Sondra felt mounted, along with a sense of gloom about why her life wasn't working out the way she'd planned. These difficult feelings soon become overwhelming, and Sondra would inevitably end up self-medicating with sugary foods. Over time, this shrunk her brain, making her less able to choose healthy emotional responses.

As I shared with you in the Introduction, I myself have turned to sugar for its soothing power. As long as it's only an occasional choice, I think it's perfectly fine to have a cookie. Eating one cookie isn't going to instantly turn you into a food addict or shrink your brain overnight.

Because Sondra wasn't getting all the nutrients she needed, however, and because she had never changed her addictive attitudes and behaviors, she had remained vulnerable to food addiction. She might escape them when times were good, but she fell prey to them again when times were hard.

Sondra's challenge was all the more difficult because, of course, food is everywhere. Unlike a substance abuser, she couldn't simply avoid the places where she had once gotten high. She was always going to find brain-shrinking foods in her break room at work, in the store on her corner, at her family's Sunday dinners, at her boyfriend's apartment. All the places she might have gone to escape the bad influences of a drug habit were places that beckoned and tempted her to indulge her food habit. As I tell my patients, food is the most socially acceptable drug of choice, making it all the harder to overcome a food addiction and keep our relationship to food inbounds. With the impulsivity associated with a shrunken brain, it can feel nearly impossible to say no whenever a trigger is encountered.

The Dangers of Tolerance

One of the key hallmarks of an addiction is *tolerance*: when you keep needing *more* to get the same high. As we build up tolerance to addictive substances, they don't have the power to give us the same kick they once did. Not only do we need more to get the same high, eventually we need them just to feel normal. Thank your brain for keeping you safe. It's adjusting and regulating its output of neurochemicals for you. If your brain kept on pumping out the same amount of dopamine and serotonin every single time you consumed sugar and bad fats, you'd have an even more serious problem on your hands—and in your brain.

You can see this quite clearly with a caffeine addiction. First you drink a cup of coffee and get a pleasant buzz. You feel a bit more alert and awake for a couple of hours.

Then one cup of coffee barely has any effect, so you up your dose to two. Then eventually you need three, and the buzz isn't quite as powerful. Your brain has adjusted its output to protect you. Pretty soon you're drinking coffee several times a day, just to stay awake. From a mild and pleasant stimulant, caffeine has become the only thing standing between you and utter exhaustion.

The same thing happens with addictive foods:

First you just enjoy them.

Then you need them. You still enjoy them . . . but it hurts not to have them.

Then you need them desperately, just to feel normal. You might not even enjoy them anymore—but you know you feel lousy without them.

Is it possible to have just an occasional brain-shrinking food and *not* get hooked? Sure! The Scripps study rats who were fed sweet, bad-fat-filled foods for only an hour a day never made the switch to becoming addicted. Their brains continued to work as they always had because their exposure was not great enough to trigger any change. (Likewise, if you limit your intake of caffeine to healthy limits, you'll probably keep getting a sustainable energy boost when you do drink coffee or tea.) And, the study that proved the existence of sugar brain didn't find that eating sugar and bad fats once instantly shrinks the brain. It was the people who were eating these foods around the clock who were the most likely to have shrunken brains.

Rats in the Scripps study that had unlimited access to those bad-fat-filled foods, however, developed tolerance. The more they ate, the less they felt it. That's why they couldn't stop eating and why they couldn't stop gaining weight.

ADDICTION PRESCRIPTION

Why can't we simply regulate our brain chemistry through medication? Couldn't we take something to prevent outside stimulants from throwing our brains out of balance?

People with substance-abuse problems frequently get substitute drugs. Heroin addicts receive methadone, smokers use Nicorette, and alcoholics and other drug users are prescribed anti-anxiety drugs—all to help wean them off their primary drugs more slowly. The substitutes blunt or prevent withdrawal symptoms, allowing people to clear their systems and rebalance their brain chemistry without suffering.

Well, guess what? In the Sugar Brain Fix program, we're following the same effective principle! I'm going to have you detox from addictive foods *gradually*, as you fill your diet and your life with Mediterranean foods and keto-inspired practices that boost your supply of healthy brain chemicals naturally. That way you can overcome your addiction painlessly and transition effortlessly into a healthy new life.

Making It through Withdrawal

Besides tolerance, the other hallmark of addiction is *withdrawal*—the pain of giving up an addictive substance that the body has come to rely on. In my private practice, I've treated people who were addicted to any type of drug, food, or behavior you can think of. I know very well how painful the recovery process can be.

Here are some of the most common withdrawal symptoms; they plague addicts to food, nicotine, alcohol, and drugs all pretty much equally. Have you noticed any of these symptoms whenever you've tried to change *your* diet?

- problems with memory
- impaired concentration
- changes in sleep patterns
- anxiety
- depression
- fatigue
- increased reliance on other addictions
- moodiness
- irritability
- headaches

Sound familiar? No wonder it's so hard to let go of our favorite treats! And as you now know, many of these symptoms will only get worse as your brain shrinks. We're used to thinking of dieting as an emotional issue or a matter of willpower, and those certainly may be elements in our struggles. But at the same time, you're suffering from profound physical symptoms and from the negative emotions inevitably generated by your unbalanced brain chemistry. Why *wouldn't* you self-medicate those symptoms with your favorite treat?

If a steady diet of sugar and bad fats could keep you feeling good, it might be worth risking the weight gain, heart disease, diabetes, and cancer that you're putting yourself at risk for, as well as whatever negative feelings you have as the result of your struggles with weight. Unfortunately, because of tolerance and withdrawal, food addiction is not a stable solution to the problem of unbalanced brain chemistry and a shrunken brain. You're always going to keep wanting more, and you're always risking withdrawal symptoms the moment you cut back. It's hard to revel in the pleasures of food when food feels like your jailer.

Addiction and Yo-Yo Dieting

Suppose, like my patient Sondra, we do make it through two weeks of chemical detox from our diets of sugars and bad fats, however painful or unpleasant that might be. Suppose, like Sondra, that we've done that not only once but twice, three times, maybe up to a dozen times as we went from diet to diet to diet. Each time we lasted one month, maybe two, maybe even six, making it well past the withdrawal symptoms and maybe even dropping a few pounds. But sooner or later we find ourselves turning to foods with tons of bad fats and sugar, and our diets fail. We're right back to shoving brain-shrinking foods into our mouths.

Once again, brain chemistry is the culprit. We need to maintain healthy serotonin and dopamine levels to feel good, and if we aren't eating the right foods or engaging in the right activities, our levels will fall too low. We may force ourselves to forgo our "medication" for a few weeks or even a few months. But unless we genuinely learn to replace it with something healthier, we'll always be tempted to come back. As our brain shrinks, the temptation grows.

ARE YOU "NATURALLY" FAT?: THE TRUTH ABOUT GENETICS

Can you be "naturally" fat? The answer is both yes and no.

Yes, up to one-third of the factors that determine body weight can be attributed to our family inheritance. Studies of twins and adopted children have revealed that biological relatives tend to be a similar body weight, even if they grew up in completely different households. First-degree relatives of moderately obese people (50 to 60 pounds overweight) are three to four times more likely to become obese than people from a different type of family. First-degree relatives of severely obese people (90 to 100 or more pounds overweight) are five times more likely to develop obesity. At least some of this correlation seems to be genetic rather than having to do with family eating habits and emotional patterns.

But no, regardless of what anyone else in your family looks like, you don't *have* to be obese, and you don't have to starve yourself to stay thin, either. What you eat, how you exercise, and how you nourish your brain chemistry through both food and activities all play an enormous role in determining your metabolism and your weight. That's because you can switch these genes off by changing what you eat and how much you move.

In 2010, genetic researchers in the United Kingdom studied more than 20,000 people who were between 39 and 79 years old. Their conclusion: Thirty minutes of moderate exercise per day can reduce any genetic tendency toward obesity by 40 percent. Other studies have come to similar conclusions.

So here's the bottom line: Regardless of who's in your family, if you follow the Sugar Brain Fix and learn how to grow your brain, you're well on your way toward achieving your healthy weight, especially if you make exercise a regular part of your day. And guess what? The right kinds of moderate exercise will also feed your brain chemistry, boosting your levels of both serotonin and dopamine, along with fasted workouts that boost brain-growing BDNF. Now that's what I call a win-win!

Getting to Know Your Hunger

I hope you can see by now that if you're at an unhealthy weight, you're responding to brain cues that have nothing to do with your body's need for nourishment.

One of the best ways to address body, brain, and emotion together is to get in touch with your hunger, which is one of the first things I ask my patients to do. I'm going to ask the same of you.

I'd like you to ask yourself the following questions each time you feel hungry. Don't judge or blame; just notice.

When do I feel hungry?

—after something upsetting happened

—after something wonderful happened

—because I'm bored

—to take a break

—when I feel like I deserve a reward

—based on a cue: after a TV show is over, when I get home, etc.

How do I feel hungry?

—suddenly I'm ravenous

—gradually, my hunger goes from being a small feeling to a progressively greater one

—I crave particular foods or types of food

—I feel desperate

—I feel calm and pleasant anticipation

—I am constantly hungry

—I am constantly looking forward to my next meal

—I look forward to the food itself

—I look forward to some other aspect of the meal: the break, the time with family or friends, the chance to get away from work or out of the house

None of these responses is wrong or bad, though some of them might be signs that your body, brain, or spirit isn't getting something that it needs. Feeling constantly hungry, for example, probably means that you're not nourishing yourself properly, whether you're overly restricting your diet, eating too much sugar (creating blood sugar spikes of "fullness" followed by crashes of feeling ravenous), or otherwise not correctly feeding your brain chemistry. It could also mean that there is a huge emotional hunger in your life that isn't being met—but, as we've seen, that is a brain chemistry issue as well as a physical one. It could also be that with a shrunken brain, change feels too difficult.

If we're eating healthy meals filled with brain-boosting foods, usually we'll feel gradual hunger every two to three hours. The diet in this book is filled with foods that keep you fuller for longer periods of time. Intermittent fasting teaches many people to undo the pairing of the slightest twinge of hunger with a sprint toward the fridge. Every time you teach yourself to tolerate a feeling that feels foreign and uncomfortable, you're on your way to making that feeling feel normal and comfortable. Fiber from vegetables and good fats from fish or walnuts ensure the food moves slowly. You can start listening to the signals for physical hunger from the hypothalamus—not the emotionally charged memories from the hippocampus and amygdala. If we've stuffed ourselves with a big meal, we may not feel physically hungry for at least six hours, as physical hunger usually comes on slowly and gradually. However, as we've seen, if you've been under stress and your cortisol levels have risen, you are likely not to feel hungry as you cope with the problem that stresses you. Then, when the stress is over—when the deadline is met or the baby finally stops crying—you may feel ravenous. That is also a physical response, triggered by your body's response to a stress hormone, but it doesn't necessarily indicate that you need food.

Eating when you're bored, to give yourself a break, on a set schedule, or in response to a cue might mean that you're eating food you don't really need. One study compared Americans to French eaters, showing that the French are more inner-directed when it comes to hunger, listening to their bodies rather than to social cues. Americans, by contrast, ate according to external cues. For example, we tend to stop eating when the TV show we're watching is over or when others have stopped eating.

As you can see, sorting out how, when, and why you feel hungry and how you might best respond is a complicated business, and there are no simple rules or easy answers. However, what will help break the hold of your food addiction is just to notice when, how, and why you feel hungry. Notice your body, your emotions, your schedule, and the cues you might be responding to. Don't judge, blame, or expect yourself to do something; just *notice*.

We'll come back to this question of hunger and your body's cues as we move through the four weeks of the Sugar Brain Fix. Later in the program, when you've added serotonin- and dopamine-boosting foods and activities to your diet and your life, you may notice places where you'd like to make a change. You might even notice that, naturally and gradually, a change has already taken place.

GASTRIC BYPASS AND LAP-BANDS: ARE THEY THE ANSWER?

Lap-Bands and gastric bypass surgeries work by physically altering the stomach's capacity. You become unable to eat more than a tiny amount at any sitting, perhaps as little as a small carton of yogurt. If the only problem with out-of-control eating were your capacity to fill your stomach, a gastric bypass or Lap-Band would work well.

The problem is that just restricting your access to food doesn't change the reasons that you were eating excessively in the first place. If your brain chemistry remains unbalanced—if your brain is still jonesing for dopamine and serotonin—keeping yourself from eating too much at one time will not change the dynamic. People who need weight-loss surgery also tend to have shrunken brains from years of eating sugar and bad fats, so they're more likely to feel blue, stuck, impulsive, and foggy. Thus, they need tools to address these states.

Certainly, these surgeries help save lives. Many morbidly obese people have benefited from them. But in my professional opinion, surgery alone is not enough. If you're considering this procedure, be sure to also use cognitive behavioral tools and self-hypnosis to help you deal with your emotional connection to food and rewire your brain.

In fact, most patients are noncompliant with at least one of the behavioral changes recommended within one year of having bariatric surgery. Many either do not exercise or do not adhere to the recommended changes in diet. I have treated a number of patients who have had these surgeries and have regained all the weight they lost initially. When this is true, they are putting themselves at risk for complications and can stretch their surgically modified stomachs.

If you're considering either of these procedures, start preparing your mind before you change your body. Go see a therapist for at least a few months to figure out whether there are any options besides surgery or, if you decide surgery is the best option, how to prepare yourself emotionally. Don't fall into polarized thinking, where you see only a single either/or choice. If you choose surgery, it's vital to combine it with other strategies to be successful.

Bear in mind that after surgery, you're going to be getting less serotonin and dopamine from food than you did previously. That makes it all the more important to follow the diet and lifestyle suggestions in this book, and that you make sure to get more of your feel-good chemicals from booster activities so that you are relying not only on food to keep your brain healthy.

The Reward Response

There is one other aspect of addiction I'd like you to know about. We've seen that sugary foods relate to our hunger for serotonin and that foods filled with bad fats feed our need for dopamine. But whenever anything pleasurable happens to us—from receiving a compliment to eating a healthy meal to enjoying a decadent dessert—we also get a little shot of dopamine, a tiny burst of *Yes! That feels good!*

That little bit of dopamine serves as a reward for anything we do that feels good. As you can see from the examples I've chosen, it can be a reward for good behavior or bad, for a healthy choice or an unhealthy one. It's simply our body's way of acknowledging that something felt good—whether that good feeling is "good for us" in the long run or not.

Many of us have struggled with relationships that we know aren't always good for us but that sometimes *feel* good at the time, even if we know there's going to be a price to pay later. When that unavailable or unreliable hottie smiles at you or asks you out, it might feel so good that you're willing to ignore your awareness that he might not show up or that she might let you down later on. That little shot of dopamine often feels so good that it's hard to imagine feeling low later.

Likewise, when a sweet or fatty treat beckons and we take that first bite—or sometimes just *imagine* taking that first bite— we get that little dopamine rush, and it feels wonderful. We can try to picture what comes later, when we feel bloated, frustrated, or annoyed with ourselves, but our present reality is that brain chemical, which gives us an immediate, powerful reward.

This dopamine reward is one of the reasons addictions are so hard to give up, even when we've physically detoxed from them. As we saw earlier, just looking at or imagining a sweet treat can set up powerful responses in our brain, with dopamine kicking in at the very thought of the pleasure we can expect. Even when the physical addiction is broken—when there are no more withdrawal symptoms and our brain has regrown—that dopamine reward beckons, and it can be very hard to resist.

What's the solution? Giving yourself so many other rewarding, nourishing activities and so many healthy dopamine boosters in your diet that those unhealthy choices are no longer your only or your primary source of dopamine-fueled pleasure. When your body and your brain really feel as though you're living in a world of plenty, your addictive responses simply become less interesting and maybe, eventually, not interesting at all. The solution is not to fight them or blame yourself for having them, but to notice them and learn about them while adding all sorts of other pleasurable choices into your life.

The bigger your brain, the easier it is to keep making good choices. That's what the Sugar Brain Fix is all about—and that's why it works.

Chapter 4

THE SECRET OF GRADUAL DETOX

When Marisa strode into my office, I felt I was in the presence of a force of nature. Short, dark-haired, and intense, she rattled off a series of rapid-fire sentences in a firm, no-nonsense tone. You could tell that this co-founder of a rising new financial services company was used to making things happen—and fast.

Marisa nodded intently as I explained to her the nature of food addictions and the relationship between her brain chemistry and her struggles with weight. But when I shared with her my approach to gradual detox, she balked.

"What do you mean I'm going to spend two weeks adding healthy new foods into my diet before I even begin to cut out the bad foods?" she sputtered. "I don't have time to screw around, Dr. Mike. I'm a very disciplined person. Just tell me what to do, and I'll do it."

I could see that Marisa's drive and determination—enormous assets in her business life—were actually getting in the way of her personal development. She had already told me that she'd tried three previous weight-loss plans, each of which had failed. I had the feeling that with all three of them, she'd flung herself into a wildly disciplined regime with a kind of cold-turkey approach to food detox. Then, when crises hit, she didn't have the resources to handle them. Her superior discipline crumbled, she returned to all her favorite comfort foods—and then, when her schedule eased up, she looked for another diet.

I didn't want to be one more failure on her list. More important, I wanted to give *her* the chance to create a lasting transformation.

"Marisa," I said, trying to find the words that would get through to her, "you told me that last year you quit smoking. Did you do it cold turkey?"

She looked at me with surprise. "Of course not. I took Zyban. Even then it was tough—but I did it. I do everything I set my mind to."

"That's terrific," I told her. "And I'm glad you gave yourself so much support and boosted your dopamine while you were trying to give up nicotine. That's exactly what I'm trying to do with your addiction to food. We need to give you lots of support, build up your healthy habits, and ease the pain of withdrawal. That's what gradual detox is all about."

Marisa stared at me in astonishment, then made one of her characteristic quick decisions. "Fine," she said, opening her arms wide in a gesture of surrender. "Let's get started."

What Is Gradual Detox?

As I explained to Marisa, gradual detox is a way of slowly letting go of an unhealthy habit by gradually replacing it with something else, allowing you to circumvent the possibility of withdrawal. One obvious example of gradual detox is when smokers use nicotine gums or patches, or when they take Zyban or other medications. These approaches blunt the agonies of withdrawal either by tapering off nicotine intake slowly or by helping to restart the production of dopamine and other brain chemicals that cigarette smoking has undermined.

Likewise, with the Sugar Brain Fix program, I'll keep you from feeling any withdrawal symptoms by having you continue to eat the brain-shrinking foods you crave. As we've seen in previous chapters, addictive foods inhibit your body's ability to manufacture its own stores of serotonin and dopamine, which, over time, shrinks the brain. As a result, when you stop eating them, you feel uncomfortable withdrawal symptoms and crave the addictive foods even more. When you feel blue, stuck, and anxious—all effects of a shrunken brain—it can feel almost impossible to resist or change your ways.

✓ With gradual detox, you'll never feel a single withdrawal symptom. That's because you'll be adding new foods, activities, and thought patterns to your daily routine, so that you'll have restored your body's ability to manufacture its vital brain chemicals. Omega-3s, amino acids, vitamins, and minerals in foods from the diet you'll eat during the Sugar Brain Fix support serotonin and dopamine production. You'll grow your brain with more BDNF from fasted workouts. That way, when you begin to cut back on the addictive foods, your body will be getting all the serotonin and dopamine that it needs. A bigger brain will help you to feel happier and less impulsive. Gradual detox makes the transition from addiction to freedom feel easy and even pleasant.

Did you know it takes at least 10 exposures to a new healthy food to accept and then to crave it? That's why the Sugar Brain Fix has you adding so many healthy foods to your diet over the 28 days of the program. You're giving your body time to gradually detox from pepperoni pizza and start to crave salmon, to gradually detox from cookies and doughnuts and start to crave blueberries and spinach. The saturated fat, flour, and high-omega-6 oils in pepperoni pizza, cookies, and doughnuts shrink the brain. The omega-3s, amino acids, antioxidants, vitamins, and minerals found in salmon, blueberries, and spinach keep the brain in tip-top shape. Replacing the old unhealthy cravings with healthy new ones will happen gradually and naturally, so that you never experience withdrawal and you never feel deprived.

Gradual detox is based on the understanding that it takes a month for the human brain to create a habit. So during the 28 days of the Sugar Brain Fix, you'll be creating healthy new habits—habits that you'll start to cultivate long before you have to give up any of your unhealthy old habits! The five-minute walk in the middle of your workday or the lunch break at that healthy café will become habitual parts of your everyday life. You may be surprised how self-hypnosis can rewire the brain, making these changes easy to incorporate. The bigger your brain, the easier the changes are to maintain.

Pitfalls and Boosters

Gradual detox is accomplished through the two cornerstones of the Sugar Brain Fix: *pitfalls* and *boosters.*

Pitfalls are the foods, activities, and thought patterns that ultimately shrink your brain by lowering your supplies of the brain chemicals you need to feel happy, healthy, and energized. A pitfall food—something filled with sugar and bad fats—temporarily lifts your serotonin or dopamine levels, but the high is soon followed by a crash, and, as we've seen, these foods undermine your body's ability to make its own stores of these vital brain chemicals and will shrink your brain over time.

A pitfall activity is any type of behavior that likewise lowers your stores of vital brain chemicals and shrinks your brain. As we saw in the previous chapter, high-stress situations can boost your levels of the stress hormone cortisol, which contributes to lowered serotonin and dopamine. Low levels of serotonin and dopamine are linked to depression, and depression can shrink your brain just like sugar does. A long, boring meeting at work, an unpleasant lunch with a highly critical family member, or an ongoing relationship with someone who doesn't treat you well might all be pitfall activities, lowering your stores of serotonin, dopamine, or both. While you might not always be able to avoid pitfall activities, you can at least be aware that they call for extra brain-chemistry support to undo their damage.

We'll take a closer look at pitfall thought patterns later in the book. These are often hard to recognize as pitfalls, especially if we're used to having them. But if you can let go of your mental pitfalls, you might be amazed at how much better you feel—and at how much better your life becomes.

Boosters are the opposite of pitfalls—they're foods, activities, and thought patterns that boost your stores of serotonin and dopamine and grow your brain, giving you the physical and emotional nourishment that your body, mind, and spirit crave. The Sugar Brain Fix diet contains high amounts of anti-inflammatory omega-3s, amino acids, vitamins, and minerals that keep the brain healthy. If one day's diet includes organic, no-sugar-added yogurt, berries, salmon, and fresh vegetables, you have spent that day taking good care of your brain, helping yourself feel calm, optimistic, and energized.

Activities can also boost your brain chemistry. Whenever you take a brisk walk, spend five minutes meditating, chat with a friend on the phone, or learn something new and interesting, you are likewise boosting your serotonin and dopamine levels while keeping your brain big and beautiful. Do a fasted workout and you'll boost BDNF, which can help you to supercharge all this brain growth.

Thought patterns can further boost your serotonin and dopamine stores, setting you up for optimism, self-confidence, and joy. In Chapter 14, I'll help you identify seven booster qualities that you can use to replace your seven pitfall thought patterns.

There are two steps to this process:

1. First add booster foods and booster activities to your life.

2. Then gradually reduce pitfall foods and pitfall thoughts.

That's it. It's that simple. Fill your life with foods, activities, and thought patterns that grow your brain, and you'll find it remarkably easy to let go of the pitfall foods and thought patterns that have been setting you up for a shrunken brain, food addictions, and excess belly fat. Once your life is full of boosters, you'll have a much easier time eliminating the pitfalls—and you'll notice how easy it is to keep your waistline trim and your brain big and beautiful.

Why the Sugar Brain Fix Works Where Other Diets Fail

If you're like most people, pitfall foods are a part of your everyday life, keeping you addicted and coming back for more as you shrink your brain. I'm sure by the time you've picked up this book, you've tried not once but many times to limit your calories or portions—but to no avail. If you're like the vast majority of people, you've been on diet after diet, all of which have failed in the long run.

Why don't diets work? Because, as we've seen in previous chapters, they didn't free you from your addiction to pitfall foods or focus on foods and activities that grow your brain. You'll notice that there's no strict calculation of carbs or daily calories in this program. Why? Because that's an approach from the outside in that imposes an external limit upon you. To make matters worse, it doesn't address the withdrawal that you're likely to feel if you try to cut back on pitfall foods abruptly, without addressing your brain chemistry. You'll go right back to those brain-shrinking foods.

To make matters still worse, the outside-in approach is doomed to fail in the long run because, without addressing food addiction, you're going to keep longing for pitfall foods that temporarily boost serotonin and dopamine levels. You may be able to resist those longings when things are going well, but when stress or major challenges inevitably reenter your life, you're likely to turn to the old reliable pitfalls that pull you deeper into addiction. The more your brain shrinks over time, the harder it is to change.

What's the result? You feel hopeless, decide you're a failure, and berate yourself for your lack of willpower. This pitfall thinking keeps you trapped in the downward spiral of sugar brain. More addictive foods that release serotonin and dopamine. A brain that keeps shrinking and a waistline that keeps expanding. The more the brain shrinks, the more you'll tend to feel blue, stuck, impulsive, or foggy. Eventually, it makes change feel almost impossible.

The Sugar Brain Fix, by contrast, works from the inside out. I want you to let go of pitfall foods *only when you feel ready to do so.* That's why I haven't even suggested cutting anything back during the first 14 days of the program. Keep eating sugar, flour, pro-inflammatory soybean oil, grains, and fried foods. I'll go further—I don't *want* you to cut back. Just add in booster activities and up your fruit and vegetable intake. All the vitamins and minerals you'll be consuming will help your body to convert amino acids into feel-good serotonin and dopamine, and it's a potent way to begin shifting from a pro-inflammatory to an anti-inflammatory diet. The letting go of your old ways of eating, thinking, and feeling will practically happen by itself.

Adding food to your diet will tackle the root of sugar brain. Tackle food addiction through boosters that will help you balance your brain chemistry. You can improve your mood by eating omega-3- and amino-acid-rich foods. You can also shred fat and increase BDNF with a little intermittent fasting paired with fasted workouts. The boosters will also help you to improve your life as you grow your brain. You'll have the body, the brain, *and* the life you want.

When you've completed the Sugar Brain Fix, you'll notice that your addictive cravings to eat brain-shrinking foods will have subsided. Suddenly, adhering to any dietary restrictions will be doable, because you've worked from the inside out. Since you're now feeding your brain chemistry and growing your brain, you'll probably find yourself wanting to eat less in general. Your body has recalibrated to normal levels. Nothing will be off limits forever, because, as the research shows, occasional exposure to pitfall foods doesn't cause addiction or instantly shrink your brain. Not to mention that saying *"I'll never eat sugar again"* sometimes can make you want it more!

The Sugar Brain Fix: 28 Days of Gradual Detox

How does this work in practice? Let's take a look. Here's the basic outline of 28 days of the Sugar Brain Fix.

WEEK 1

Don't cut any foods out of your normal diet. We add before we take away.

Eat at least *seven* servings of whole fruits and vegetables. These will ensure you're getting the vitamins and minerals needed to manufacture serotonin and dopamine while keeping your brain big and beautiful.

Eat at least *one* omega-3-rich food every day. This will ensure you're getting more brain-boosting, anti-inflammatory, good fats.

Skip or replace *one* breakfast or dinner this week. You can either skip the meal altogether or replace it with bone or vegan broth.

Do *one* fasted-state workout. This is a workout done just before the meal that comes after the one you skipped or replaced. Most people prefer to do cardio in the fasted state, but you can do any type of moderately rigorous exercise for a minimum of 30 minutes.

Add *one* boosting activity each day. Based on your findings from the quizzes in Part II, I'll give you a list of activities that will replenish the neurochemicals you need most. If you need to replenish both serotonin and dopamine, alternate by adding a serotonin booster one day and a dopamine booster the next.

WEEK 2

Don't cut any foods out of your normal diet.

Eat at least *seven* servings of whole fruits and vegetables. These will ensure you're getting the vitamins and minerals needed to manufacture serotonin and dopamine while keeping your brain big and beautiful.

Eat at least *one* omega-3-rich food every day. This will ensure you're getting more brain-boosting, anti-inflammatory, good fats.

Skip or replace *two* meals this week. You can either skip these two meals altogether or replace them with broth. Skip or replace one dinner and the next morning's breakfast, or skip or replace two nonconsecutive meals: one breakfast and one dinner; two breakfasts; or two dinners.

Do at least *one* fasted-state workout. Work out just before a meal that comes after one you have skipped or replaced. Most people prefer to do cardio in the fasted state, but you can do any type of moderately rigorous exercise for a minimum of 30 minutes.

Add *two* serotonin- or dopamine-boosting activities each day. As with your food boosters, if you're deficient in both serotonin and dopamine, add one booster activity for each neurochemical every day.

WEEK 3

Limit your pitfall foods to no more than *three* servings per day. A pitfall food serving should be around 300 calories at most, so you're going for a maximum of about 900 calories from foods made with brain-shrinking sugar (in all its forms) and bad fats.

Eat at least *seven* servings of whole fruits and vegetables. These will ensure you're getting the vitamins and minerals needed to manufacture serotonin and dopamine while keeping your brain big and beautiful.

Eat at least *one* omega-3-rich food every day. This will ensure you're getting more brain-boosting, anti-inflammatory, good fats.

Skip or replace *three* meals this week. Skip or replace one dinner and the next morning's breakfast plus one additional breakfast or dinner. If this is too difficult, you can skip or replace three nonconsecutive meals: three breakfasts; three dinners; two breakfasts and one dinner; or one breakfast and two dinners.

Do at least *two* fasted-state workouts. Work out just before a meal that comes after one you have skipped or replaced. Most people prefer to do cardio in the fasted state, but you can do any type of moderately rigorous exercise for a minimum of 30 minutes.

Add *three* serotonin- or dopamine-boosting activities each day. If you need to replenish both types of brain chemical, alternate between adding two serotonin boosters and one dopamine booster, and adding one serotonin booster and two dopamine boosters.

WEEK 4

Limit your pitfall foods to no more than *two* servings per day. Remember, one serving of a pitfall food is about 300 calories, so you're looking at a maximum of about 600 calories of foods made with brain-shrinking sugar (in all its forms) and bad fats.

Eat at least *seven* servings of whole fruits and vegetables. These will ensure you're getting the vitamins and minerals needed to manufacture serotonin and dopamine while keeping your brain big and beautiful.

Eat at least *one* omega-3-rich food every day. This will ensure you're getting more brain-boosting, anti-inflammatory, good fats.

Skip or replace *four* meals this week. Skip or replace one dinner and the next morning's breakfast—and do this twice this week. Or, skip or replace one dinner and the next morning's breakfast plus two additional nonconsecutive breakfasts or dinners. Or, skip or replace four nonconsecutive meals: four breakfasts; four dinners; or a combination of breakfasts and dinners.

Do at least *two* fasted-state workouts. Work out just before a meal that comes after one you have skipped or replaced. Most people prefer to do cardio in the fasted state, but you can do any type of moderately rigorous exercise for a minimum of 30 minutes.

Add *four* serotonin- or dopamine-boosting activities each day. If you need to replenish both types of brain chemical, add two boosters of each type every day.

MAINTENANCE

Follow the program you followed in week 4.

LOOKING FOR A SHORTCUT?

I'd like you to read every word of this book because I think the more you understand about the way foods affect your brain, the more empowered and proactive you'll be at implementing the Sugar Brain Fix and making it work for you.

But if you're eager to get started and just want to know exactly what to do, here's how you can move through this book more quickly:

- Take the quizzes on pages 65 and 91 in Part II. They will help you figure out whether you are serotonin deficient, dopamine deficient, or both.

- Based on what you learn about your body chemistry, go to the lists of booster foods and activities on pages 190, 191, 202, and 203. Choose as many as you can and prepare to add them to your daily diet and lifestyle.

- Look at the outline on page 52. Select the correct number of meals to replace or skip and fasted workouts to add over the 28 days.

Those are the basics. Add booster foods and activities, intermittent fasting, and fasted workouts, gradually increasing them over the next 28 days, and, two weeks into the program, start cutting back on the pitfall foods that shrink your brain until you're down to only two or fewer servings per day (one pitfall serving is about 300 calories, so you're down to a maximum of 600 calories in pitfalls).

Fine-Tuning Your Brain Chemistry

Now that you understand the basic principles of sugar brain and the ways you can fix it, it's time to get specific. Let's move on to Part II, where you'll find out which of your brain chemicals need boosting and exactly what you need to do to boost them.

But first, we're going to hear a success story from my mom, Carol!

SUGAR BRAIN FIXED: CAROL'S STORY

They say the true test of believing in something is if you would you recommend it to your own mother. My answer: absolutely! So, I put my mom on the 28-day Sugar Brain Fix program. Since I knew we've both eaten in similar ways through our lives, I knew it was likely she also had a shrunken brain. If she could shred fat, she'd feel better and become healthier.

My mom was excited about it. She had recently lost weight after months of following a points-based program, but she was stuck at a plateau—not an uncommon phenomenon among people using some form of daily caloric restriction. I had achieved incredible results after fine-tuning the Kediterranean template of The Sugar Brain Fix, so I was confident it would work.

I signed my mom up to get a Bod Pod—a capsule-like body composition measurement machine—to get an accurate reading of her weight, muscle mass, and body fat. As you know, less fat on the body is linked to having a bigger brain. If her muscle increased while fat decreased, it was also likely she was boosting levels of the growth hormone BDNF—which grows the same part of the brain that sugar shrinks.

After she completed the 28-day Sugar Brain Fix program, I got this e-mail from my mom:

"George and I had Chinese today. We skipped the egg rolls, rice, and wontons. We ordered lots of veggies and a veggie soup."

Here's what else she noticed:

- I've lost weight. My clothes are fitting better and I'm now buying a size 14. I used to be a 16. Progress.

- Fasting isn't as hard as I thought it would be.

- I'm making better choices—not perfect, but better.

- My posture has improved noticeably. I'm drinking way more tea and water.

- I'm sleeping like a baby.

- I made a new friend at the pool.

- I put the Activity app on my Apple Watch.

- I'm actually looking forward to my measurement on the Bod Pod. I'm not expecting a miracle, but I already feel better.

Of course, she is my mom—so admittedly, she's biased. So, let's look at her unbiased results.

BEFORE THE SUGAR BRAIN FIX

DATE: 6/7/18
WEIGHT: 174.8 lbs.
BODY FAT: 77.6 lbs. (44.4%)
LEAN MASS: 97.2 lbs. (55.6%)

AFTER THE 28-DAY SUGAR BRAIN FIX

DATE: 7/8/18
WEIGHT: 170.6 lbs.
BODY FAT: 72.7 lbs. (42.7%)
LEAN MASS: 97.9 lbs. (57.3%)

AFTER ANOTHER MONTH—FOLLOWING THE SUGAR BRAIN FIX **MAINTENANCE** PROGRAM

DATE: 8/7/18
WEIGHT: 165.9 lbs.
BODY FAT: 67.5 lbs. (40.7%)
LEAN MASS: 98.4 lbs. (59.3%)

TOTAL NUMBER OF POUNDS LOST: 8.9
TOTAL NUMBER OF POUNDS OF BODY FAT SHREDDED: 10.1

THE TAKEAWAY: In just a few months, my mom lost a significant amount of weight. But perhaps more importantly, she shredded fat while *gaining* muscle. This is probably because the one change in her exercise routine was adding weight-based interval training as her fasted workout—which was an addition to her usual routine of swimming. If you can't afford body composition testing, know that sometimes the number on the scale may not change very much—or not at all. But if you're following the program, you're probably shredding fat even if the number on the scale doesn't change. If you have the time and funds to get this type of testing, do it. Bod Pods or dunk tanks (another way to accurately measure body fat) usually cost between $25 and $50 per session.

As a free alternative, I have included a weekly waistline measurement in your 28-day journal. If this measurement decreases by even the smallest amount, you have done something incredible for the health of your brain—not to mention your body.

My mom's reported improvement in mood was a clue that she was likely improving her serotonin and dopamine levels with booster activities.

Today, I can see the differences in the way my mom eats. When I was home for the holidays, she snacked on roasted veggies in olive oil. This was a big step in the right direction from our family's go-to "vegetable" I remember from our childhood: broccoli casserole—a little broccoli with bad-fat-filled cheese and crushed saltines on top. I see her drinking water and stevia-sweetened sodas instead of aspartame- or sucralose-sweetened ones. My mom looks and feels better. I'm proud, and I worry less about her health.

Part II

YOUR BRAIN ON THE WESTERN DIET

Chapter 5

FEELING ANXIOUS

Hungry for Serotonin

As we saw in Part I, serotonin is a key brain chemical that's crucial for many mental and physical functions. This peace-giving substance soothes, comforts, and encourages. High levels of serotonin make us feel optimistic and hopeful about achieving our goals and triumphing over our challenges. Low stores of serotonin make us feel anxious, fearful, and pessimistic about what we can accomplish.

Serotonin's importance to our brains is best illustrated by the cases of people with severely low levels. People with a history of aggressive behavior such as arson, assault, and murder have been found to suffer from drastically low serotonin levels. Self-directed violence, including self-mutilation and suicide, has also been associated with low serotonin. On a less extreme level, low serotonin has been linked to obsessive-compulsive behavior, chronic pain, chronic digestive problems, alcoholism, sleep disturbances, chronic fatigue syndrome, migraines, cluster headaches, and eating disorders.

So when you're feeling anxious, upset, or despairing—especially when you're hungry—this is not a sign of poor character or emotional weakness. You are experiencing your body's desperate need for serotonin. The solution is not to berate, restrict, or question yourself. The solution is to feed yourself! Your body, mind, and spirit will all benefit from the booster foods and activities that you'll add when you follow the 28-day plan of the Sugar Brain Fix. And you'll be amazed that, maybe for the first time in your life, you no longer feel hungry, but full, content, and at peace.

Are You Hungry for Serotonin?

In my personal and my clinical observation, the vast majority of people in the United States are serotonin deprived, which is why sugary foods have such a hold on us. Our culture is fast-paced, and our obsession with following mostly frightening or disturbing news all day long only feeds the uncertainty that most of us feel. People are much more likely to live alone than in decades past, and this can lead to increased feelings of loneliness. A working parent may feel held hostage by constant worry—especially if he or she is the only parent actively involved in the child's life. But there is a solution.

The first step in solving the problem is identifying the problem. If we can find out what is missing from your life, then we can also figure out what we need to add to your life, so you can get the serenity, hope, and peace you deeply crave. Once we target these underlying emotional issues through booster activities and foods that support steady levels of serotonin production, you may be relieved to discover that your battle with food no longer feels like a constant struggle. So let's take that first step and find out what's going on with your brain chemistry. Take the following quiz to find out if low serotonin is an underlying cause of your sugar brain.

GET THE FULL PICTURE

Whatever your results, please don't stop here. You might *also* be ravenous for dopamine. Whether you score high or low on the serotonin quiz, check out the next chapter to make sure you've gotten the fullest possible picture. You need both scores to choose the version of the Sugar Brain Fix that is perfect for *you*.

Are You Hungry for Serotonin?: A Quiz

Score the following:

0—never   2—sometimes   4—always
1—rarely   3—frequently

1. I feel that I'm not getting enough of one or more of the following: cuddling, serenity, peace, or quiet.

2. When I feel blue, my idea of comfort might include one or more of the following: seeing a therapist, meditation, yoga, a gentle stroll, a romantic movie, peaceful music, or talking to someone to cheer me up.

3. I enjoy tea or wine.

4. When I'm in a bad mood, I crave sugar; foods with a soothing texture, such as ice cream, or soothing temperatures, such as soup; or familiar foods.

5. I don't like it when things are out of place.

6. I don't like it when people are late.

7. I question myself and wonder whether I'll be good enough to reach my goals.

8. I often wonder why other people seem to have it so much more together than I do.

9. I often feel lonely.

10. I prefer a job where there is not much pressure or where I can work alone without competition, demands, or high risk.

11. I like to take care of others by cooking.

12. I will eat when others do, just to be polite.

13. I startle easily or am easily frightened.

14. I often get stuck in anxious thoughts.

15. I'm fearful.

16. I carry a lot of tension in my body, especially my neck, back, shoulders, around the temples, or in my jaw.

17. I get migraines or frequent headaches.

18. When I have a physical symptom, I worry about what potentially life-threatening disease I might have.

19. I have trouble falling asleep.

20. I don't like to sit still. I either pace, do something with my hands, or have something in my mouth. I rely on gum, toothpicks, cigarettes, candy, knitting, playing with my hair, or some other way of keeping busy.

21. I often feel nervous.

22. I often have the feeling that things are not going to be okay.

23. I eat to calm myself down.

24. I often feel overwhelmed.

25. I don't like change.

26. I consider myself a conflict-avoider or people-pleaser.

27. When things are bad, I have trouble seeing any hopeful possibilities.

28. I have a history of anxiety, panic attacks, obsessive-compulsive disorder, anorexia, agoraphobia, or phobias. (If no, score this item 0; if yes, score this item 4.)

Scoring

Total from item 28 _____

Now, multiply this number by 3.

x3 = _____ (A)

Add up your scores for items 1–27.

Total: _____ (B)

If you are a woman, put a 5 in box C.

If you are a man, put a 0 in box C.

_____ (C)

A + B + C = _____ (D)

Your score: _____

DID JUST TAKING THIS QUIZ MAKE YOU FEEL ANXIOUS?

If it did, don't worry. That's a perfectly normal reaction—especially if you're starved for serotonin—and it doesn't mean that anything's wrong. It only means that your default reaction to stress is to feel anxious.

The good news is that whatever your score, there is something you can do about it—something that won't be difficult and that might even be fun. Remember, *gradual detox* means that you get to keep eating everything you already enjoy while adding serotonin boosters to your diet and your life. Adding these new foods and activities will go a long way toward calming your anxieties and making you feel great. So take a slow deep breath, release it slowly, and then read on to find your score.

Are You Hungry for Serotonin?: Your Score

0–20: Satisfied and at Peace

Congratulations! Your serotonin levels are healthy, and you've figured out how to keep them that way. Your balanced brain chemistry is paying off with a feeling of well-being, self-confidence, and peace. Read the rest of this chapter to understand how you can identify your mantra and other key elements of the Sugar Brain Fix. Then move on to Chapter 6 to explore whether you are ravenous for dopamine.

21–36: Hungry for Serotonin: Moderate, Frequent Anxiety

If you scored in this range, your anxiety is under control, but it's a far greater presence in your life than it needs to be. You may be aware of your anxiety as something that impedes your pleasure, or you might be so used to feeling anxious that you don't even think about wanting to feel less so. Again, the good news is that you can start taking steps to make yourself feel better by undergoing gradual detox from the foods and thought patterns that are contributing to your anxiety. Read on through the rest of this chapter to find out more.

Over 36: Famished for Serotonin: Moderate to Intense Anxiety, Almost Always

If your score was over 36, your serotonin levels have fallen very low, and you are understandably desperate to feed them. You probably experience frequent, intense cravings for brain-shrinking sugars, and you may also struggle with mood swings that are linked to when and how you eat. You may be frustrated, discouraged, or despairing about how out of control you feel, both of your moods and your appetite. Please don't berate yourself any longer. You are simply doing your best to feed your brain chemistry, but you haven't yet been given the tools to help you do that in a way that does so while growing your brain. Now you have those tools: The Sugar Brain Fix will help you rebalance your brain chemistry without making you feel deprived. Congratulate yourself for starting this journey. Read through this chapter for concrete, specific suggestions that will start you on your healing journey.

Note: If you scored anything but a 0 in box A, or your total score was 40 or above, I strongly recommend that you work with a health-care professional to implement the Sugar Brain Fix. Your program may require additional support. See Appendix B on page 309 for more details.

Serotonin and Your Body

If you've just found out that you're serotonin deficient, you might begin to see what has perhaps been behind a host of issues you've struggled with. Low serotonin causes emotional ailments such as anxiety, depression, and lack of self-confidence. It can also cause such physical disturbances as trouble with sleep, digestion, and pain. Serotonin is crucial not just for our brains but for our entire bodies.

For example, together with melatonin, serotonin is central to our ability to fall asleep, to stay asleep, and to sleep deeply. We often crave sweets late at night, which may be our body's way of seeking the natural sleep assistance of this crucial brain chemical. The problem is that the same sweets that help us fall asleep work the same way that drinking alcohol before bed does. Both may cause drowsiness, but in the long run, they actually prevent you from getting the deep sleep you need to feel rested and alert the next day. They can help you *fall* asleep, but using these foods as your sleeping aid may also lead you to wake up in the middle of the night when the "high" wears off. Healthy, stable supplies of serotonin are crucial for good sleep.

Digestion relies on serotonin, much of which is manufactured in the gut. Serotonin helps our abdominal muscles contract so they can push food through the gastrointestinal tract. Low serotonin may be associated with a variety of digestive problems, including irritable bowel syndrome.

Finally, serotonin is a known pain reliever. That's why when our levels are low we often feel achy and more easily laid low by any type of physical challenge. This is also why serotonin-boosting antidepressants are prescribed for chronic pain, even if the patient doesn't report depression.

I don't want you to worry about these potential maladies, but I do want you to understand: If your stores of serotonin are low, it is very difficult for you to function in a healthy, relaxed way. Eating sugar is an understandable response to this uncomfortable state. Unfortunately, if you try to feed your serotonin-starved brain with sugar, you'll only make the problem worse. First, because of the tolerance element in addiction, you'll need more and more sugar just to get the same comfort.

Second, because of withdrawal, you'll feel terrible any time you try to give up sugar. You reached for addictive, brain-shrinking foods in the first place because you thought they would make you feel better—and they do, temporarily. But they also con-spire to make you feel worse, particularly when you are holding on to or gaining weight.

What's the solution? First, add healthy serotonin boosters to your diet and your life. Then, gradually, when you're getting all the serotonin you need, you can slowly reduce the number of pitfall foods that you were once relying on as a serotonin crutch. At the same time, as we'll see in this book, you can begin to replace pitfall thoughts with boosters—positive, supportive ways of thinking that will also help your serotonin levels rise.

SUGAR'S SWEETNESS GOES BEYOND TASTE

The brain-stimulating effects of sugar are so addictive that mice whose ability to taste sugar had been removed still chose sugar water over regular water every time they were presented with both. Clearly, neither taste nor "psychology" were involved. The mice were responding purely to the chemical effects of sugar.

How to Make More Serotonin *Without* Sugar

There's a healthy way to get more serotonin from the food you eat. Now that you've learned how sugar floods the brain with an instant hit of serotonin while shrinking the brain, let's look at how healthy foods help you maintain a steady supply of serotonin while simultaneously keeping your brain big and beautiful.

Serotonin can be made from the amino acid tryptophan, found in many healthy foods. Unsurprisingly, diets low in tryptophan have been shown to increase anxiety. This, of course, can fuel cravings for foods with brain-shrinking sugar to self-medicate. Let's look at a very simplified diagram of serotonin and how your body converts tryptophan in your diet into the chemical 5-HTP, which is then converted into serotonin.

TRYPTOPHAN → 5-HTP → SEROTONIN

So, just eat more tryptophan, right? Well, not quite, because your body struggles with this conversion without certain vitamins and minerals needed to activate the chemical process. Folate, vitamin B_6, vitamin C, zinc, and magnesium are all needed for optimal serotonin production. Let's look at how these vitamins and minerals from foods you'll find in the Sugar Brain Fix diet facilitate the process:

> TRYPTOPHAN (FROM EGGS) → FOLATE (FROM SPINACH) → 5-HTP → VITAMIN B_6 (FROM SALMON), VITAMIN C (FROM RASPBERRIES), ZINC (FROM CHICKPEAS), AND MAGNESIUM (FROM CASHEWS) → SEROTONIN

Without enough of these healthy foods, you may also have trouble sleeping since serotonin metabolizes into melatonin. Without sufficient sleep, you're likely to crave more brain-shrinking, sugary foods the following day.

To ensure you'll be getting the vitamins and minerals that support serotonin production, you'll eat seven servings of vegetables and whole fruits every day as part of the Sugar Brain Fix. The average American eats only about three per day. Bonus: The antioxidants that are found in vegetables and whole fruits help protect your brain from shrinking by combating oxidation, which, like sugar, can shrink the brain. And the fiber found in vegetables and whole fruits will help you to feel full.

The proof that this makes a difference you can feel? In 2013, a study of more than 80,000 people found that those who ate seven servings of vegetables and whole fruits per day were happier, less nervous, and had higher levels of life satisfaction and well-being.

In Chapter 12, I'll share a complete list of serotonin-boosting foods that contain tryptophan, vitamins, and other minerals that your body needs to make serotonin naturally.

Why Artificial Sweeteners Are Also Bad for Your Brain

Sucralose (Splenda), aspartame (Equal), saccharin (Sweet'N Low), and acesulfame potassium or acesulfame-K (Ace-K, Sunett, Sweet One) are bad for both your brain and your waistline.

A 2017 analysis of 37 different trials and studies found that consumption of artificial sweeteners was associated with increases in weight and waist circumference in humans. And as you know, a larger waist is linked to having a smaller brain.

The question remains: If artificial sweeteners have no calories, how or why would they be linked to an expanded waistline? New research offers answers to this question.

Consuming artificially sweetened foods and drinks may affect how much and what you eat. Research has found that animals fed artificial sweeteners will start to consume larger quantities of foods, and the foods tend to be sweet, calorie-dense ones. When researchers stopped feeding them artificial sweeteners, the animals stopped eating all the extra, sweet food.

Although they're not metabolized like sugar, artificial sweeteners can also negatively affect your brain via the gut-brain connection. Most of your serotonin is manufactured in your gut and then travels to your brain. Artificial sweeteners have been shown to kill the gut bacteria that manufacture feel-good neurotransmitters like serotonin. Just like not having enough of the amino acids, vitamins, and minerals depresses serotonin levels, not having enough good gut bacteria decreases levels of this feel-good neurotransmitter. If serotonin levels are low, you're more likely to crave sugar—since it floods the brain with serotonin.

But research shows that's just the first thing that happens. Through this connection between artificial sweeteners and your gut, artificial sweeteners can later affect your blood sugar levels. Rats were fed artificial sweeteners at levels that would be equivalent to what's been deemed an acceptable level in humans by the Food and Drug Administration. A control group did not consume artificial sweeteners. Later, all the rats were given a sugary drink. Rats who had been consuming artificial sweeteners had blood sugar levels that spiked higher *and* took longer to drop back to normal. As you might expect, having blood sugar levels that spike and stay high is a recipe for sugar brain.

In addition to changing the way your body responds to sugar, research has shown that artificial sweeteners affect the way you respond to fat. A 2018 study found that artificial sweeteners can change the way you metabolize food. Rats were given either sugar or artificial sweeteners. Sugar negatively impacted the rats' ability to burn fat, which, of course, can lead to both weight gain and sugar brain. Surprisingly, the artificial sweeteners had the same effect as sugar—interfering with the rats' ability to burn fat. Yet it *also* negatively affected the rats' ability to create energy.

Part of the Sugar Brain Fix diet template is all about revving your metabolism with mild-ketosis-promoting, fat-burning tools. Keeping blood sugar low for most of the day is essential to grow the brain and bust belly fat. We now know artificial sweeteners may interfere with this process. To fix your sugar brain, eliminate or reduce your use of artificial sweeteners.

Sleep, Serotonin, and Insulin Resistance: How Sugar Makes You Tired and Hungry

As we have seen, sweet, starchy foods toy with you like a seductive, unreliable lover. One minute, they're promising to satisfy all your cravings. The next minute, they've left you hungrier than ever.

The reason for this roller-coaster appetite is insulin resistance. Insulin is a hormone made in your pancreas that transfers glucose (blood sugar) from your bloodstream to your cells. We call it blood *sugar,* but that's a misleading term. Blood sugar rises or falls in response to everything you eat: fat and protein, as well as sugar.

However, sugar causes your insulin levels to spike because sugar, flour, and fruit juice metabolize quickly, dumping a lot of sugar into your blood at once. Insulin will then flood your system because it's trying to bring down those high blood sugar levels by transferring that sugar into your cells.

If your insulin spikes too often, your cells will eventually begin to adapt by reducing their response to insulin, which then leaves the glucose floating aimlessly in your bloodstream. Your blood sugar is too high, and your cells aren't getting enough of it. Your pancreas will initially respond by making more insulin to saturate your insulin receptors, but over time the pancreas will start to reduce the amount of insulin it releases.

This is a recipe for diabetes and exhaustion. And most paradoxically, it also leads to a constant appetite, since your sugar-starved cells are sending hunger messages to the brain, unaware that all the sugar they need is right there in your bloodstream.

Significantly, serotonin levels rise as you eat, helping your brain to register when you feel satisfied. So if your brain is low on serotonin, it won't understand that you're "full," and you're likely to keep eating, even when your body has had enough. Besides making you feel anxious, low serotonin levels make you more likely to overeat and less likely to feel satisfied. That's why you often crave dessert, even when you feel "stuffed" and understand intellectually that you are no longer hungry. And, of course, we all know that lethargic feeling we get when indulging in too much food, commonly known as a "food coma."

Over the long term, the weight you gain from your serotonin shortage can lead to all sorts of problems. You gain weight and develop sleep apnea, which in turn can lead to restless sleep and sleepiness during the daytime. Once again, you're caught in the downward spiral of using food to make up for this general feeling of low energy, even as the food you choose depletes your energy further.

The solution? Gradually replace serotonin *pitfalls* like sugars with serotonin *boosters*: foods and activities that help keep your serotonin at a nice, stable level. If you don't reverse this downward spiral, you're setting yourself up for serious health problems, including sugar brain. It's very difficult to simply feed your serotonin addiction "a little" and remain "a little" overweight. Due to the nature of tolerance, you're going to crave ever-increasing amounts of sugar, and your weight—as well as all the related health risks—will continue to increase. Another part of the solution is to add intermittent fasting to help improve insulin levels and sensitivity. Unlike caloric restriction, our diet helps with insulin resistance.

The good news is that if you can turn this situation around, you'll create the opposite effect. Every healthy change will give you the energy to make more changes, which will make you even healthier.

Why Dieting Makes You Miserable— Especially If You're a Woman

Americans quickly embraced no-carbohydrate diets, and now when people want to lose weight, cutting back on carbs is usually what they try first. Twenty years ago, it was Atkins. Today, it's strict, traditional keto. But doing so can dramatically affect your brain chemistry, especially if you're a woman.

Researchers at the Massachusetts Institute of Technology found that carbohydrates cause the brain to release serotonin. Without enough sugars to perform this crucial function, dieters become serotonin deprived and may feel anxious, irritable, and depressed. In one study, animals deprived of tryptophan—a key amino acid used to make serotonin—became far more aggressive. Now we can see that when dieters have a similar reaction, it's not a character weakness but a biological response.

Women and those under ongoing stress may be the most at risk. Why? They tend to be sensitive to changes in serotonin. Depressed women have been shown to respond more favorably than men to antidepressants that target serotonin, suggesting that low serotonin levels are indeed a significant problem for women and one that makes ordinary diets very problematic for most.

We know that women are about twice as likely to be diagnosed with depression as men, and they're also far more likely to suffer from migraines. Serotonin is likely responsible for a great deal of that discrepancy. Whether women lack serotonin because of their inherent biology or because they face social stressors and negative conditioning that men are spared, the result is the same: Most women are at a serotonin deficit that can easily become a serious problem if either new stress or a restrictive diet further depletes their stores.

Researchers in another study found clear evidence of women's special difficulties with diets. After three weeks on a low-calorie diet, men and women had lost a similar amount of weight. However, the women were left more anxious and unhappy and far more vulnerable to mood swings than their male counterparts. If the diets had offered women alternative sources of serotonin, the women might have lost weight *and* felt better.

Meet Your Mantra: A Powerful Tool for Self-Transformation

As we've seen, low serotonin levels produce anxiety. But it works the other way, too: Anxiety and other forms of stress deplete your serotonin.

ANXIOUS THOUGHTS → LOWER SEROTONIN LEVELS → MORE ANXIOUS THOUGHTS → EVEN LOWER SEROTONIN LEVELS → MORE ANXIOUS THOUGHTS . . .

Does the problem start with anxious thoughts or lowered brain chemistry? No doctor can pinpoint exactly how it started for you, and it doesn't really matter. Once you start on that downward spiral, you'll keep going unless you do something deliberate to interrupt it. You need to either change your thoughts or boost your serotonin levels—or both.

Combining sources of tryptophan with vitamins and minerals from vegetables and fruit can boost serotonin levels. As you'll see in Part IV, your 28-day Sugar Brain Fix will add serotonin boosters to your diet in a more systematic way.

But there is also quite a bit you can do to replace pitfall thoughts, which generate anxiety, pessimism, and low self-confidence, with booster thoughts, which generate peace, optimism, and confidence. In Part IV, you'll learn how to identify the seven pitfall thought patterns associated with bad moods and poor eating habits. But before you learn how to specifically target and transform these negative thought patterns, you'll work with a global and powerful thought-transforming tool: your *mantra*.

Your mantra is a brief but powerful statement of your core belief about yourself and the world. Booster mantras improve our brain chemistry by creating a positive, abundance-based, and confident approach to life. Pitfall mantras, which are negative, make us more likely to turn to addictive foods, alcohol, or drugs, thereby keeping us anxious, pessimistic, and discouraged. The more you avoid the pitfall styles of thinking you'll learn in Part IV, and the more you add the booster attributes to your life, the easier it will be to move from a pitfall mantra to a booster one. Likewise, the more you work on transforming your mantra, the easier it will be to avoid pitfall thinking and bring booster attributes into your life.

Self-medicating with food only makes a pitfall mantra worse and can lead to a downward spiral if the "medicine" you're choosing is an addictive pitfall food. The "sugar high" is inevitably followed by a "sugar low," just as the temporary calm of noodles and white bread gives way to an anxiety and hunger that are even more intense than before. You *can* lift your mood with booster foods and activities. In Part IV of this book we'll find out how. But I'd also like to help you get at the thoughts and feelings that exacerbate your anxiety in the first place.

The key to this is understanding your pitfall mantra and then replacing it with a more positive message. This will interrupt the cycle of anxious thoughts and free you from its downward spiral. A positive booster mantra will allow you to feel better about yourself, your life, and your future even before you've reached your healthy weight.

Sound good? Then let's get started. The first step is to identify your mantra.

Identifying Your Mantra

If you're struggling with low serotonin, your current mantra is likely to reflect anxiety, pessimism, and a lack of confidence. Here are some common "hungry for serotonin" mantras:

Something bad is going to happen to me.

If I don't do something in one exact way, something bad will happen.

If that could happen, then anything could happen.

If I'm not a complete success, I'm a complete failure.

If I don't weigh myself frequently, my weight might balloon.

If I don't control my feelings, I'll fall apart completely.

If I ever let anyone down, I'm a complete failure as a person.

If others get close to me, they'll hurt me.

Do any of these sound familiar? If one of these statements perfectly describes the way you think about yourself and the world, look no further. You have found your pitfall mantra. Go right ahead to the next section to find out how this mantra affects your weight.

But if none of these statements quite hits the nail on the head, take a few moments to articulate your own personal pitfall mantra. It's worth spending a little time on this because I want you to be able to recognize this way of thinking the moment it rears its ugly head. And believe me, it will. One thing I've learned from both my own growth and that of my patients is that as soon as we start making positive changes, all the old pitfall thoughts and feelings from the past rush up to try to pull us off track. If you can recognize your pitfall mantra, you'll be far more effective at transforming it into your new booster mantra.

So grab a notebook and a pen, or sit for a moment at your computer, and write down your own personal pitfall mantra. What words do you keep hearing that make you feel anxious, unworthy, or pessimistic? Write them down, look at them for a moment, and then move on to the next section.

How Your Mantra Affects Your Weight

Your pitfall mantra might be different from mine, but they definitely share one thing in common: Each time we repeat our pitfall mantras, our serotonin levels drop.

When you're hungry for serotonin, pitfall mantras lead to anxious pitfall behaviors, and those pitfall behaviors cause serotonin levels to drop, too. Whenever we behave in a fearful, anxious way—obsessing over every bite of food or extra ounce of weight or refusing dates until we've lost those last 10 pounds—we reinforce our fearful attitudes and lower our serotonin.

This interaction between brain chemistry and experience goes back to our childhoods. Say you come from a stormy, argumentative family with a father who was always exploding in rage and a mother who was known for her frequent criticisms. As a child, you may often have felt fearful and anxious, afraid that your slightest error might provoke your parents. This state of fear would have helped to "set" your serotonin at a chronically low level. These same low serotonin levels would contribute to your anxious state.

But it doesn't stop there. Your anxious feelings might then drive you to choose fearful actions such as hanging back from the other kids at school or not wanting to leave the house until your outfit is perfect. These fearful actions in turn reinforce the idea that the world is dangerous (the kids will mock you, your outfit will make you look bad), leading you to become still more cautious. The combination of anxious thoughts and fearful behavior continues to drive down your serotonin levels. And now we have all the elements of a vicious cycle, in which attitudes, behavior, and brain chemistry all work together to keep you anxious and miserable.

SEROTONIN LEVELS → MORE ANXIOUS THOUGHTS
→ FEARFUL ACTIONS → REINFORCING STRESS
→ EVEN LOWER SEROTONIN LEVELS → MORE
ANXIOUS THOUGHTS . . .

No wonder serotonin deficiency creates cravings for brain-shrinking foods! When you're feeling anxious and fearful, you're more likely to reach for sugar that temporarily eases your mind by boosting your serotonin levels. You're starving for anything that will make you feel better, and food may feel like the only comfort you can rely on.

Transforming Your Mantra

Now that you've identified your old pitfall mantra and seen how it affects your life and your weight, let's change it into a new, more positive statement about yourself and the world. For example, if your core belief is *I'm not safe*, I'm going to give you the tools to change it to a more optimistic message, such as *Everything is fine*. Here are some of the booster mantras you might choose:

I'm a resourceful person and can handle the things that come up.

Things will turn out okay . . . they usually have before.

I'm good at many things, and if a few things aren't perfect, that's okay.

I do what I can . . . and I'm okay with that.

I've done my best . . . and my best is pretty good.

Even when things are hard, I can imagine that they will get better.

Look over these improved mantras and see if one of them works for you. If so, write it down. We'll be coming back to it again later. If none of these is perfect for you, take a few moments and create your own. You deserve a booster mantra that expresses exactly the attitude and core beliefs by which you choose to shape your life.

How Your Sugar Brain Fix Will Transform Your Mantra

Maya was a teenage girl who struggled with her weight. Her parents were both fit, successful attorneys. Maya, on the other hand, weighed close to 200 pounds. Her parents' high standards and fit bodies made Maya feel like a failure, as did their well-intentioned efforts to stock their kitchen with Maya's "special diet food." So when her parents weren't home, Maya would medicate her loneliness by eating boxes of cookies in the middle of the night.

Maya was a junior at a prestigious private school, where she had good friends—but no dates. She compensated for her weight by buying expensive clothes. But I saw, too, that her mantra, "No one will ever truly love me for me," was preventing her from allowing any guy to get close. And covering up who she really was with all these accoutrements was exactly what prevented her from being seen, known, and loved.

Together we labeled all of her pitfall styles of thinking. But no amount of logical discussion was going to change the fact that no boy had ever asked her to a high school dance. Nothing we said was enough to make Maya feel pretty or love her body. And until she did feel good about herself, she would never have the stores of serotonin she needed to give up the sugar that she used to medicate her misery.

"I know that logically I *should* feel good enough," Maya told me once. "That doesn't change the fact that I still *feel* sad and just awful about myself. I know I'm smart, but I keep comparing my life with other people's. Being at the top of my class doesn't really feel like it's worth very much. Honestly, if I could trade my intelligence to be 60 pounds lighter, I would. I have friends that love me, but I've never had a boyfriend. And every time I try on clothes I *feel* terrible about myself, and then nothing else that's good in my life seems to matter."

What Maya was saying to me—and what perhaps you are now saying to yourself—is that words and logic aren't enough to change our feelings. In order to create a new mantra, you must give yourself new experiences. You must try out some new actions and pay attention to the consequences, and allow those consequences to affect you.

Here are a few simple examples. Do any of these speak to feelings that you recognize?

Old Belief	New Action	New Consequence	New Belief
I have to be perfect.	I did something imperfectly every day this week.	Nothing terrible happened.	Maybe it's okay not to be perfect *all* the time.
I am not lovable.	I smiled and said hello to a stranger five times this weekend.	Two people ignored me, but three people smiled and said hello back.	Maybe there is something good in me that people can love.

The power of transforming core beliefs is at the heart of the Sugar Brain Fix. Adding self-hypnosis to the mix makes the changes in what you do and how you eat feel even easier. Signing up for a class on a topic that has always intrigued you, getting in touch with old friends, treating yourself to a massage or a manicure, joining a social or political group, reaching out to ensure you have support in your life—all of these are new booster actions that will improve your brain chemistry, open you to new consequences, and allow you to really start believing your new mantra. Now we've transformed a downward spiral into an upward spiral:

BOOSTER ACTIVITIES → POSITIVE CONSEQUENCES
→ BOOSTER THOUGHTS → MORE SEROTONIN → MORE
SELF-CONFIDENCE, OPTIMISM, AND PEACE → MORE
ENERGY FOR MORE BOOSTER ACTIVITIES → POSITIVE
CONSEQUENCES → *MORE* BOOSTER
THOUGHTS → *MORE* SEROTONIN . . .

That's the payoff of the Sugar Brain Fix. Transforming and maintaining your new mantra may take a while, and you may experience some ups and downs along the way. But you can make a significant change in only 28 days, and after that, the momentum of the upward spiral will help keep you on your path. Just start by adding a few booster foods and activities. Supported by a new, more positive mantra, you may be amazed at what happens next.

Boosting Your Belief in Yourself

One of the mantra-related challenges I give my patients is the "Because . . ." exercise. I ask them to pick a positive statement about themselves that they know logically to be true, and to come up with as many reasons as possible for *why* it is true. For example:

I *am* okay because:

. . . I love my mom.

. . . I'm a friendly person.

. . . my life has potential.

. . . I like where I live.

. . . my ability to sing makes me happy.

. . . I know I am a good person inside.

Sometimes I ask my patients to carry this list with them and to find at least three items to add to it throughout their day. I also ask them to reread it before every meal. These booster thoughts genuinely nourish the brain chemistry and affect how you feel and what you're hungry for. Why not give it a try? It's forcing you to put on what I call the "what's right" glasses: You're training yourself to look for the real and omnipresent evidence that supports your new mantra.

Do You Have the Happiness Gene?

Without even meeting you for a diagnosis, I can tell you the answer to this one: No. *Because there isn't one.*

Just as body weight isn't determined solely by genetics, neither is happiness. In both cases, there is an interaction between genetics, life experience, and personal choices that helps to shape our outlook as well as our bodies.

True, some of our potential for happiness *might* be contained in the levels of serotonin, dopamine, and other brain chemicals for which we are coded. Some of us are born with naturally higher ranges of those chemicals than others, and this can make a difference in our personalities, outlook, and general sense of well-being.

It's also true that our life experience affects our brain chemistry, especially during childhood. Those of us who grew up in anxious or angry households are likely to have gotten used to lower levels of key "feel-good" chemicals than people from calmer and more supportive households.

However, neither of these factors is enough to determine our destiny. As we've seen throughout this book, the decisions you make every day—choosing booster or pitfall foods, activities, and thoughts—have a profound effect on how you feel. Your biological or childhood inheritance may give you some bigger challenges to overcome, but it is absolutely within your power to create a happy, peaceful, and satisfying life.

Satisfying Serotonin

When you begin your 28 days of the Sugar Brain Fix, you'll be working to boost and balance your serotonin levels. For the first two weeks, you won't cut back on anything, but you will feed your body and your spirit with lots of serotonin-boosting foods and activities.

As you begin to make new, healthier food choices, be sure to arm yourself with information. Part of why sugar is so hard to avoid is because it's *everywhere*—even in foods you probably thought didn't have any. Sugar, high-fructose corn syrup, and other addictive sweeteners are added to bread, "unsweetened" cereal, ketchup, fruit juices, and many other foods that you probably never thought of as "dessert." The foods you do think of as sweets may also contain far more sugar than you imagine.

When you start to feel positive reinforcement—in the form of people noticing you've lost weight, your own glances at the mirror, and your improved energy and mood—it will be easier to continue transforming your mantra into a positive and life-affirming one. Your cravings for sugar will vanish, and your blood sugar will remain on an even keel. You'll feel hungry periodically, not constantly, and your food will satisfy you. And if you still desire an occasional treat, go ahead! Enjoy yourself! When your serotonin levels are high, everything about your life—including dessert—just feels better. Your mantra, your diet, and your brain chemistry will all support your going forward to create the life you were born to live.

Chapter 6

FEELING BLUE

Ravenous for Dopamine

When you're feeling anxious and fearful, you're hungry for serotonin. But when you're sad, lonely, or listless, you're ravenous for dopamine.

Dopamine is the brain chemical associated with thrills and challenges. When we ski down a mountain, go out on a romantic first date, or visit a foreign country for the first time, our dopamine levels rise. We feel that rush of excitement that makes life seem truly worth living.

Dopamine comes mostly from anticipation—more the thrill of the chase than the satisfaction of winning the race. It's the chemical that pushes us to seek out sex, and it's what fuels our feelings of being in love. Those first, hot three months of passion? That's dopamine. (The slower, steady warmth of a loving marriage? That's serotonin along with oxytocin, the "bonding chemical.") No wonder dopamine makes us feel so good!

When our dopamine levels are healthy, life seems fun and interesting, and we are frequently tingling with excitement. When our dopamine levels are low, we tend to feel listless and blue, trapped in a boring, dead-end life.

SUBSTANCES OR BEHAVIORS THAT CUE OUR BRAINS TO RELEASE DOPAMINE

- caffeine
- cocaine
- driving fast
- falling in love
- gambling
- hunting
- nicotine
- red meat
- sex/sexual desire
- shopping (not the mundane kind, but the kind known as "retail therapy")
- participating in sports, especially extreme sports
- stock trading
- taking risks
- video games
- watching an exciting sports match

Dopamine is also released with just 20 minutes of moderate exercise.

Lack of dopamine can also make us feel unmotivated. It becomes harder to focus on long-term goals, to defer gratification, and to muster the patience for a long, hard slog to the finish line, whether it's a project at work or a demanding emotional situation.

Low dopamine levels can send us rushing for quick-fix foods and behaviors, partly because we don't have the mental, biochemical resources we need, and we know that a treat filled with bad fats or a stimulating behavior will give us at least temporary relief from our brain-chemistry blues. Foods with bad fats cue our brains to release unsustainable amounts of dopamine, giving us a chemical rush of excitement and pleasure. So we keep on eating those foods while shrinking our brains.

You might end up dopamine deficient for a number of reasons. Perhaps your recent life circumstances have been constricting, boring, or enervating. Lack of sleep and stress can also cause a dopamine deficiency, which is why you often crave fat more when you're feeling tired or under pressure. Or maybe you're coming down from an intense, thrilling period—a passionate affair or a series of challenges—and you're feeling the crash. You might have inherited a tendency to lower dopamine levels or developed them through a childhood marked by high-stress and high-risk situations, such as when children grow up with an addicted or mentally ill parent, or parents who are prone to rage, tantrums, or abuse. While this type of high-stress childhood can also deplete serotonin levels, it sometimes creates a kind of roller-coaster emotional ride for children, who get "hooked" on the adrenaline-fueled challenge of high-stakes crises, such as how to calm an out-of-control parent or how to cope with financial turmoil.

Another possibility is that, like the rats in the Scripps study, you have harmed your dopamine-pumping neurons with a diet filled with bad fats. You may have overwhelmed your brain's ability to process the chemical, which often leads to lowered natural production.

Any type of dopamine deficiency leaves us feeling low and listless, so that we naturally turn to bad fats that will perk us up. Once again, we're trapped in a downward spiral that ends with a shrunken brain:

> LOWER DOPAMINE LEVELS → LISTLESS FEELINGS → EATING MORE BAD FATS → DAMAGE TO NEURONS WHILE THE BRAIN MAKES LESS DOPAMINE → EVEN LOWER DOPAMINE LEVELS → MORE LISTLESS FEELINGS → EATING MORE BAD FATS → MORE DAMAGE TO NEURONS WHILE THE BRAIN MAKES EVEN LESS DOPAMINE → EVEN LOWER DOPAMINE LEVELS . . .

In the previous chapter, we saw how low serotonin levels were connected to anxiety, pessimism, and lack of self-esteem. Low dopamine levels can lead to their own set of pitfall attitudes that soon manifest themselves in pitfall behaviors (see the chart below). Ironically, the response to both the unpleasant feelings and the upsetting behaviors often seems to be self-medication with foods filled with bad fats. While this provides temporary relief, it also locks us even more firmly into the downward spiral.

Attitudes and Behaviors Associated with Low Dopamine Levels	
Depression	Risky behavior
Loneliness	Emotional eating
Feelings of being unlovable	Isolating oneself
Procrastination	Short attention span
Boredom	Low sex drive
Distractibility	Low work performance
Hyperactivity	Impulsive choices

Are You Ravenous for Dopamine?

Just a quick look at the mammoth portions in U.S. restaurants should be enough to tell us that, in addition to being serotonin starved, many of us are also dopamine deprived. Why else would we chase all the bad fats in fried foods, desserts, pro-inflammatory red or processed meat, and snacks such as chips? Why else would we consume so much caffeine? Why else are the airwaves full of ads for energy drinks and caffeine pills? We're all exhausted, run-down, and sleep deprived—and our eating habits show it!

I have a lot of sympathy for this one, too. I look at my patients, who are often working multiple jobs or stretching themselves to the limit trying to work a full day *and* raise a family, and I can't believe how stressed they are. We're all anxious about our changing world, a competitive global market, and we're all under pressure to work around the clock, as well as to expend enormous energy parenting our children. Many of us are working jobs we don't enjoy or feel trapped in situations that drain us. Dopamine deficiency is the result—and craving fat, caffeine, and perhaps also sugar is the consequence.

Once again, to solve the problem, we must identify the problem. So take a closer look at your dopamine levels by taking the following quiz.

GET THE FULL PICTURE

Make sure to take both the following quiz and the one in Chapter 4 to see whether you are starving for serotonin, ravenous for dopamine, or both. Your individualized 28-day Sugar Brain Fix will depend on your own personal brain chemistry, so make sure you've gotten all the facts.

Are You Ravenous for Dopamine?: A Quiz

Score the following:

0—never	2—sometimes	4—always
1—rarely	3—frequently	

1. I feel that I'm not getting enough of one or more of the following: adventure, excitement, new or stimulating life experiences.

2. When I feel blue, my idea of a lift might include one or more of the following: action movies, adventure sports, loud music, screaming, hitting

something, acting out, gambling, spending lots of money, or casual sex.

3. I often crave coffee, energy drinks, caffeinated soda, or hard liquor.

4. I often crave fatty foods; foods that are new, adventurous, or spicy; or foods that have stimulating textures, such as crunchy chips or salty popcorn, especially when I'm in a bad mood.

5. I don't mind things being out of place.

6. I often procrastinate or show up late.

7. I have gravitated toward jobs that involve risk-taking, competition, and high stakes.

8. I often find myself working with large groups of people and usually enjoy it.

9. I isolate myself and don't like reaching out when I'm in a bad mood.

10. I want things when I want them.

11. I'm not a detail-oriented person.

12. If I haven't reached my goals, that's not my fault.

13. People would say I tend to make impulsive decisions.

14. I often have trouble listening.

15. I often wonder what's wrong with other people.

16. I often can't finish things.

17. I often have trouble staying asleep.

18. I have lost interest in things I used to find pleasurable.

19. I love adventure and change.

20. I would rather say what I mean, even if it means hurting someone else's feelings.

21. I often have trouble concentrating.

22. I often feel bored.

23. I often have low energy.

24. I often feel restless.

25. I often feel hopeless.

26. I often find myself crying or tearful.

27. I often feel generally dissatisfied with life.

28. I have a history of depression or ADD/ADHD.
    (If no, score this item 0; if yes, score this item 4.)

Scoring

Total from item 28 _____

Now, multiply this number by 3.

x3 = _____ **(A)**

Add up your scores for items 1–27.

Total: _____ **(B)**

If you are a woman, put a 5 in box C.

If you are a man, put a 0 in box C.

_____ **(C)**

A + B + C = _____ **(D)**

Your score: _____

DID JUST TAKING THIS QUIZ MAKE YOU FEEL INADEQUATE?

People have that reaction frequently, because—especially if you're deprived of dopamine—you may frequently feel that you're just not measuring up, can't get the job done, or don't have the internal resources to do what you would like to do.

I want to stress that these feelings have *no* bearing on reality. Feeling inadequate is a common reaction to a dopamine shortage, and when your brain chemistry is balanced, you're likely to feel quite different. The good news is that whatever your score, there is something you can do about it, something that won't be difficult and is likely to feel good. Remember, gradual detox means that you get to keep eating all the foods you already enjoy while adding dopamine boosters to your diet and your life. These boosters will help you find the motivation to get moving, the patience to reach your goal, and the energy to get there. So shake off the sense of inadequacy, prepare yourself to take action, and read on to find your score.

Are You Ravenous for Dopamine?: Your Score

0–20: Motivated and Energetic

Congratulations! Your dopamine levels are healthy, and you've figured out how to keep them that way. Your balanced brain chemistry is paying off with a feeling of excitement and pleasurable anticipation as you look forward to your life. If you haven't already, make sure you have thoroughly read Chapter 5 to explore whether you are hungry for serotonin. Finish this chapter before moving on.

21–36: Ravenous for Dopamine: Moderate Listlessness, Impatience, or Sense of Inadequacy

If you scored in this range, your dopamine is at a moderately low level, and it's bringing you down. You are not as motivated as you would like to be, and you are frequently plagued with feelings such as "What's the use?," "I'm not going to make it," or "I don't see the point of even trying." You can find your energy and rediscover life's pleasures by beginning your gradual detox from the foods and thought patterns that are contributing to your listlessness. Read on through the rest of this chapter to find out more.

Over 36: Famished for Dopamine: Persistent, Sometimes Overwhelming Depression, Listlessness, or Fatigue

If your score was over 36, your dopamine levels have dropped to a seriously low level, and you may be desperate to bring them back up. You are likely to feel intense cravings for foods filled with bad fats, and you may also struggle with feelings of fatigue, depression, or despair that improve only when you eat. You may be worried or confused about why you can no longer access your usual energy and excitement. Please don't be concerned. Your brain chemistry has gotten out of balance, and while you might be doing your best to restore its health, perhaps you don't have the right information to help you do it effectively. Now you can take action, starting with your 28-day Sugar Brain Fix. Keep reading to find the tools you need to make an action plan.

Note: If you scored anything but a 0 in box A, or had a total score of 40 or above, I recommend that you work with a health-care professional to implement the Sugar Brain Fix. Your treatment may need to be supplemented by additional support. See Appendix B on page 309 for more information.

The Proven Way to Make More Dopamine *Without* Bad Fats

Just as you can manufacture steady supplies of serotonin from healthy Mediterranean foods, the same is true for dopamine. Now that you've learned how bad fats flood the brain with an instant hit of dopamine while shrinking the brain, let's look at how healthy foods help you maintain a steady supply of dopamine while simultaneously keeping your brain big and beautiful.

The Building Blocks of Dopamine

Dopamine can be made from the amino acid tyrosine, which is found in many healthy foods. Let's look at a very simplified diagram of dopamine and how your body converts tyrosine in your diet into L-dopa and then dopamine.

TYROSINE → L-DOPA → DOPAMINE

However, your body needs vitamins and minerals to facilitate this chemical process. Without iron, vitamin C, folate, and copper, your body struggles with this conversion. Let's look at how the vitamins and minerals from the foods you'll find in this book facilitate the conversion process, keeping dopamine high and your brain healthy:

TYROSINE → IRON (FROM SPINACH) → VITAMIN C (FROM YELLOW BELL PEPPERS) → FOLATE (FROM ASPARAGUS) → L-DOPA → DOPAMINE

The seven servings of vegetables and whole fruits you'll be eating as part of the Sugar Brain Fix will ensure you're getting enough of the vitamins and minerals that support dopamine production. When dopamine levels are steady, you're less likely to crave brain-shrinking bad fats.

In Chapter 13, I'll share a complete list of dopamine-boosting foods that contain tyrosine, vitamins, and minerals your body needs to make dopamine naturally. For now, let's look at why Mediterranean foods are such powerful sources of dopamine.

Fish, Seafood, and Other Animal Products

Along with the emphasis on vegetables and whole fruits, the Mediterranean diet emphasizes good fats with high levels of omega-3s to help fix your sugar brain and boost dopamine. The landmark study that proved the existence of sugar brain found that people who ate lots of grilled fish, the richest source of anti-inflammatory omega-3s, were more likely to have bigger brains. The people who were eating lots of burgers, high in both saturated fat and pro-inflammatory omega-6s, were more likely to have shrunken brains. So if you're low on dopamine, eat lots of clean fish. If you do eat animal products, favor ones that are higher in omega-3s—like free-range eggs and organic chicken.

Seafood is the richest source of omega-3s. Research shows that eating fish is more effective at getting omega-3s into your bloodstream than taking omega-3 supplements. If you're vegetarian, you can gobble up lots of plant-based sources of omega-3s, including walnuts, flaxseeds, and chia seeds.

Unfortunately, lots of seafood today contains high levels of pollutants like mercury. For the health of our planet, it's also important to choose sustainably caught varieties of fish. Harvard School of Public Health, the Environmental Defense Fund, and the Monterey Bay Aquarium teamed up to develop a list of go-to fish that are high in omega-3s, low in pollutants like mercury and polychlorinated biphenyls (PCBs), and sustainably caught.

Whenever possible, I recommend seafood as your omega-3-rich food for the Sugar Brain Fix. Since you'll be eating one omega-3-rich food every day, it's vital that the seafood isn't high in toxins like mercury.

Here's a list of the *omega-3 seafood superfoods*:

- Albacore tuna, troll or pole caught, fresh or canned, U.S. or British Columbia

- Arctic char, farmed

- Barramundi, farmed, U.S.

- Coho salmon, farmed, U.S.

- Dungeness crab, wild, California, Oregon, or Washington

- Longfin squid, wild, Atlantic

- Mussels, farmed
- Oysters, farmed
- Pacific sardines, wild
- Pink shrimp, wild, Oregon
- Rainbow trout, farmed
- Salmon, wild, Alaska
- Spot prawns, wild, British Columbia

While the omega-3 seafood superfoods can be expensive or hard to find, there are some affordable, portable, and easy-to-find sources at most grocery stores. Pole- or line-caught albacore tuna can be found for around $4 per can, which contains two servings. While it may be more expensive than the 99-cent cans of tuna, you get what you pay for. Pole- or line-caught albacore has about six times more omega-3s than cheaper varieties and isn't loaded with mercury. Many versions of canned wild salmon can also be found on grocery store shelves for a few dollars a serving. There's one company that ships clean, omega-3-rich seafood to your door—see Appendix B for a discount code.

When it comes to animal products, all are not created equal. The Mediterranean diet tends to have less animal protein and more plant-based protein like beans than the standard American diet. I also encourage you to add pea-protein-based foods to you diet. When you do eat animal protein, favor sources with higher levels of omega-3s by choosing animal products that are organic, grass-fed, free-range, and/or pastured. Minimize conventional and factory-farmed animal products that are high in omega-6s. Don't be afraid of good fats. Favor a small amount of organic cream over skim milk and a whole, free-roaming egg over conventional egg whites.

Grass-fed, pastured, free-roaming, and/or organic animal products also have higher levels of the vitamins and minerals that help keep your brain big and beautiful. Conventionally raised, factory-farmed animal products have lower levels of B vitamins, zinc, copper, chromium, vitamin A, vitamin C, and vitamin E.

As a consumer, you also need to be wary of the words food companies use to trick you into buying products you perceive as healthy. Unlike eggs with the words *organic* and *free-roaming*, those labeled "cage-free" or "vegetarian" may not necessarily be better for you.

A "fresh Atlantic" salmon does not necessarily mean that it's wild-caught salmon. "Vegetarian-fed" is misleading since many cheap industrial grains fed to animals that are high in pro-inflammatory omega-6s are technically plant based. But the industrial-grain diet makes those eggs higher in omega-6s. *Pastured* and *pasteurized* sound similar, but you're looking for the former when it comes to getting more omega-3s. Don't be fooled by any of the following words on animal products:

- All natural
- Vegetarian-fed
- Cage-free
- Pasteurized
- Fresh

To keep your brain big and beautiful—and to maximize dopamine's effects—what you really want to do is to get more omega-3s, so look for one or more of the following words:

- Organic
- Free-roaming
- Free-range
- Grass-fed or grass-finished
- Pastured
- Pasture-raised

The best choice of all is when you see that the words *certified humane* are included. Some food companies can get away with labeling a product as free-range if animals are given access to the outdoors. A product labeled "Certified Humane Free Range" or

"Certified Humane Pasture Raised" ensures the animals are actually spending most of their waking hours outside, where they can eat nutritious vegetation that changes the fat composition of meat, dairy, and eggs.

Grass-finished is a preferable clarification of *grass-fed*—meaning that the animal ate grass for its entire life-span. Sometimes, companies will feed the animal grass and then switch to grains and can get away with calling it grass-fed. If the food is labeled "grass-finished," that's even better.

Beans and Soy Products

Beans are another wonderful choice, since they have a favorable omega-3 to omega-6 ratio that have been shown to keep your brain healthy. While they also have some carbs, you'll be reducing your overall carb intake during your 28-day Sugar Brain Fix if you replace sugar, flour, grains, and chips with beans. Beans also have vitamins like folate and vitamin B$_6$ that help keep your dopamine levels stable. They're also inexpensive. Including more beans is also a wonderful help to our planet since it decreases your need for meat from animals.

Foods made from whole soy can also help you keep your brain healthy, but there are also some complicated caveats when it comes to soy. First, avoid soybean oil at all costs. You'll find this omega-6-rich bad fat in just about all processed foods.

In general, don't overload on soy. Cultures that have traditionally eaten soy products don't overload on them, and they tend to eat them in their natural form or fermented, which increases their health benefits. A Japanese miso soup with a few small cubes of tofu is quite different from a supposedly healthy American vegetarian diet with nonorganic, genetically modified soy-based meat substitutes at every meal. Avoid processed soy products like soy protein isolate, textured soy, vegetable protein, and soy flour, which contain cheap ingredients that food companies use to add protein or enhance texture in all sorts of different foods.

Favor pea protein over soy protein isolate. It has a wide spectrum of amino acids that can help your brain manufacture feel-good neurotransmitters like dopamine. Favor organic or non-GMO soy. Nonorganic or GMO soy has one of the highest levels of pesticides of any nonorganic food; more than 90 percent of the soybeans in the U.S. are genetically modified.

Oils

There are three types of oils you'll find in my kitchen: extra-virgin olive oil, light olive oil, and virgin coconut oil. Olive oil has been proven time and time again in study after study to be the go-to oil for a variety of health benefits. Olive oil contains high amounts of the very best type of fat—*mono*unsaturated fat. It's even better than *poly*unsaturated fat.

Get soybean oil out of your diet. This cheap oil found in almost all processed foods is the number one source of brain-shrinking omega-6s in the American diet.

While olive oil is chock-full of beneficial compounds, many people misuse it by using the same type of olive oil for cooking as they do for dressings. Extra-virgin olive oil isn't stable at high temperatures, so use it for dressings or cold salads. If you're going to heat it, look for olive oil that's labeled "light olive oil" or an ingredient label that reads just plain "olive oil." It's a great way to bring a little Mediterranean flair into your every meal, whether you're scrambling free-range eggs for breakfast or heating some frozen cauliflower rice for dinner.

Olive oil is the Mediterranean-influenced oil of the Kediterranean diet to grow your brain; coconut oil is the keto-influenced one. High-quality extra-virgin coconut oil may be safe for many people to use as a treat. Although it has high levels of saturated fat, coconut oil contains medium-chain triglycerides (MCTs), which have been shown to help people lose weight.

The Sugar Brain Fix helps you to shred belly fat, which, as you know, is linked to a bigger brain. In one study, eating a very small amount of coconut oil helped subjects to lose an inch around their waistline with no significant changes in lipid profiles.

When it comes to other oils, look to replace bad fats like soybean, corn, cottonseed, sunflower, and sesame oil. These include cold walnut oil since it contains high levels of omega-3s, macadamia nut oil, or—for high-heat cooking—Malaysian palm fruit oil. The other widely available oil you'll find is canola oil, but this oil is highly processed. Despite the fact that it contains omega-3s and high levels of monounsaturated fat, which makes it similar in composition to olive oil, these healthy fats are processed by heat, which turns the omega-3s rancid while compromising the health benefits of its fats. You may not be able to detect the rancid flavor, since some food processers add deodorizers to mask the smell. GMO giant Monsanto produces genetically modified soy and canola products that are engineered to withstand high levels of pesticides, so canola oil is also dirty and should be avoided unless it's non-GMO and labeled "cold-pressed" or "expeller-pressed."

Again, nothing beats the health benefits of olive oil, but a small amount of organic butter, ghee, or clarified butter, which have higher levels of omega-3s than conventional butter, can also be safe to eat from time to time. Consuming healthy fats can help keep your dopamine levels healthy as you wean off bad fats.

Despite big food companies' deceptive efforts, soybean oil–based vegetable spread is not "heart healthy," nor is it healthier than butter. Soybean oil contains high levels of omega-6s. Margarine and "vegetable spreads" should have no place in a healthy diet. Neither should low-calorie butter sprays made with soybean oil.

Another note about oils: Beware of the word *vinaigrette*. A healthy vinaigrette is made with olive oil and vinegar, which can reverse sugar brain. But many premade vinaigrettes are deceptively filled with brain-draining sugar and omega-6-rich soybean oil. As for mayonnaise, choose ones made from all olive oil and no soybean oil. I also love Vegenaise, which is made with expeller-pressed canola oil and isn't filled with pesticides like most sources of canola oil.

Pep-Me-Up Proteins

It's important to know that anti-inflammatory omega-3s compete for space in your cells with pro-inflammatory omega-6s. Thus, taking a fish-oil supplement can't undo all the damage of a full day of brain-shrinking, high-omega-6 foods. As you now know, animal products that are organic, grass-fed, free-range, or pastured have more omega-3s than factory-farmed varieties. That being said, organic chicken can't compare to the megadose of healthy, brain-balancing omega-3s of wild salmon.

Also, it's important to understand whether you're shifting your diet in a "less bad" or a "more good" way. Since it has less fat, conventionally raised, factory-farmed chicken breast has fewer omega-6s than conventionally raised, factory-farmed beef. If you choose the chicken over the beef, you're subscribing to a "less bad" philosophy. It's a step in the right direction—bad to fair. But to really grow your brain, you need to also subscribe to a "more good" eating plan by *adding* omega-3s. Choosing organic chicken over factory-farmed chicken takes you from fair to good. Choosing grilled arctic char, wild salmon, or pole-caught tuna takes you from good to great—a "more good" direction with lots of brain-growing omega-3s.

Plant-based sources don't provide the usable form of omega-3s your body needs. Plant-based omega-3 sources have to be converted into EPA and DHA, and your body isn't very good at this process—especially DHA. This is why vegans often take an algae-based DHA supplement. But walnuts, flaxseeds, and chia seeds are still wonderful sources of anti-inflammatory omega-3s. If you eat fish, include seafood *and* plant-based omega-3 sources in your diet.

During the 28-day Sugar Brain Fix, you'll add one omega-3-rich food beginning in week 1. Then, you'll begin limiting pitfall foods starting in week 3.

What counts as an omega-3-rich food?

- Any seafood (not fried, does not contain bad oils like soybean, canola, peanut, corn)

- While any seafood counts, I encourage you to stick to the list of omega-3 seafood superfoods since they're sky-high in omega-3s and low in mercury. Since your new template will contain more seafood, finding clean sources is vital.
- Plant-based omega-3 sources: walnuts, flaxseeds, chia seeds

Which fats/proteins count as pitfall foods?

- Anything fried
- Anything in bad oils, which includes all oils except olive, virgin coconut, cold- or expeller-pressed canola, walnut, avocado, macadamia nut, and Malaysian palm fruit
- All processed meats, including lunch meat—even white lunch meat
- All conventionally raised/factory-farmed animal products, including meat, milk, eggs, and dairy

What about organic, grass-fed, or pasture-raised milk, eggs, or dairy?

- These are "neutral" foods. While they have more omega-3s than their factory-farmed, conventionally raised counterparts, they still don't provide the hefty dose of omega-3s that seafood does. But they're not pitfall foods, either. Enjoy them in moderation.

OMEGA-6s	OMEGA-3s
Brain shrinking	Brain growing
Pro-inflammatory	Anti-inflammatory
Bad fats	Good fats
Omega-6-rich	Omega-3-rich
Western diet	Kediterranean diet of the Sugar Brain Fix

Dopamine Deprivation: Harder on Men?

I am living testimony to the fact that many people don't fit the gender stereotypes, which proclaim that men tend to be dopamine deprived while women are starving for serotonin. Speaking as a man who struggles more with serotonin issues, I know that many people do *not* align with the generalizations.

Having said that, I want to acknowledge that many studies do associate women with a craving for sweets and ice cream, while men do seem to be drawn to processed red meat, other foods filled with bad fats, and the dopamine rush of a whiskey neat. There does seem to be some biological basis for this difference, whether we're born with it, develop it in response to cultural conditioning, or a little of both.

However it came about, adult men produce more serotonin than women, and their brains store it more effectively. When men and women were subjected to the same stressors during research, eight times more blood flowed to the emotional centers in women's brains than to those of the men, suggesting that women use up their serotonin reserves more quickly than men and are more easily drained by stress. Women are about twice as likely to suffer from low-serotonin depressions than men and are also more likely to be anxious, another sign of low serotonin. Some studies show that women respond better to the antidepressants that target serotonin, suggesting that their problems lie in low serotonin levels, and their problems are eased when their serotonin levels are boosted.

Men, on the other hand, seem to be more hooked on dopamine. A 2006 study found that men are more susceptible to the effects of drugs that actively target dopamine levels. When both men and women were given doses of amphetamines, the men's brains were flooded with far more dopamine than the women's. Men are also much more likely to be diagnosed with attention-deficit/hyperactivity disorder (ADHD), also associated with low dopamine.

Some researchers speculate that men are responding to a uniquely male gene that regulates their brains' production of dopamine. Perhaps this is why men are more likely than women to develop such dopamine-related diseases as schizophrenia and Parkinson's, a condition in which dopamine-producing neurons in the back of the brain begin to die, producing the body tremors and paralysis that indicate a lack of that neurochemical.

The Dopamine Reward

If you're struggling with low dopamine, you may also have noticed a subtle way that dopamine itself acts to keep all types of addictions going. Any time we feel a sense of pleasure or the satisfaction of a craving, we get a little dopamine kick. This is true whether we're craving serotonin, dopamine, or any other brain chemical—or whether we're craving a person, an experience, an object, or a substance. Dopamine gives us a potent reward that makes it even harder to resist our cravings.

At the same time, if our dopamine levels are too low, we don't get the kick we seek from the high-fat food we turned to—and so we may continue craving fat until our dopamine levels finally rise. This relationship emerged in one study when researchers asked groups of young women to drink a milk shake while they monitored the effects it had on their dopamine levels. The women whose brain activity showed the lowest dopamine levels in the study were most likely to have gained weight when researchers met them a year later. Researchers speculated that if a woman's dopamine levels were relatively low even after a delicious milk shake, she was more likely to crave fatty foods in other instances.

What does this mean for you? If you're trying to overcome a craving for dopamine, be extra compassionate with yourself, because it may feel as though your entire body is conspiring to pull you back into the addiction. Since dopamine itself is the reward for any type of pleasure—whether satisfying an addiction or something healthier—it's hard not to want more and more and more of it. That's why I want you to be especially careful to load up your diet and your life with dopamine boosters while you are trying to let go of the unhealthy choices that are making you feel both bad and good.

Paying the Price for Your Caffeine Buzz

A key dopamine stimulator is caffeine, which some 90 percent of all U.S. adults consume daily, primarily in the form of coffee, energy drinks, and soda. Like sugar, starches, and fats, caffeine gives us a quick high followed by an uncomfortable crash. In many cases, our response to that crash is to seek either sugary or bad-fat-filled foods to pick us up again. While caffeine does suppress your appetite during the buzz, you might feel hungrier than ever when you crash.

Lack of sleep lowers both your dopamine and your serotonin levels. Caffeine can also interfere with your ability to get restful sleep, and that lack of rest lowers both your dopamine and your serotonin levels. If you're already getting less sleep than you need—and most Americans are—you may be turning to a combination of sugar and bad fats plus various forms of caffeine just to make it through the day.

What's the solution? First, get more sleep—easier said than done, I know, but crucial to your health, well-being, and weight loss. Besides decreasing your levels of vital brain chemicals and setting you up for food cravings, lack of sleep increases the production of cortisol, which cues your body to hold on to fat.

Second, take a long, hard look at how caffeine might be affecting your rest. The half-life of caffeine is six hours, which means that the coffee or energy drink you consume at 4 P.M. is leaving you with a half-dose of caffeine at 10 P.M. Even when you have no problems falling asleep, caffeine interferes with the depth of your rest. If you wake up the next day feeling tired, you're setting yourself up to crave more caffeine—and then all the sugar, starch, and fat that helps you through your caffeine cycle.

Of course, if you're drinking any of the delicious flavored coffee drinks that are so popular these days, you are most likely adding sugar and bad fats to your caffeine anyway. This combination makes these treats especially hard to resist—and also especially likely to set you up for addiction, exhaustion, mood swings, and weight gain.

In your 28-day Sugar Brain Fix, try to limit yourself to a maximum of two cups of coffee or caffeinated tea per day. You'll be engaging in activities and foods that support healthy levels of dopamine, so you may notice that excessive cravings for caffeine begin to subside. Intermittent fasting can boost adrenaline levels, so you may need less caffeine to feel awake and alert.

Low Dopamine: Frustration, Boredom, and Feelings of Inadequacy

By now you understand that low dopamine levels create listlessness, frustration, boredom, feelings of inadequacy, and, in some cases, full-blown clinical depression. But it works the other way, too: Being trapped in a frustrating, boring, or discouraging situation depletes your dopamine.

DISCOURAGED THOUGHTS → LOWER DOPAMINE LEVELS → MORE DISCOURAGED THOUGHTS → EVEN LOWER DOPAMINE LEVELS → MORE DISCOURAGED THOUGHTS . . .

Which came first, the thoughts or the brain chemistry? Like the chicken and the egg, we can't pinpoint it exactly, but it doesn't matter. What does matter is interrupting your pitfall thoughts while revitalizing your brain chemistry.

Foods that support healthy dopamine production are crucial for giving you the lift that you may now be getting from bad fats or excessive amounts of caffeine. When you get to Part IV, you'll learn how to craft your 28-day Sugar Brain Fix plan and how to add dopamine boosters to your diet every day, giving you the emotional and biochemical support you need to get off the caffeine "buzz-crash" roller coaster.

You can also harness the power of your mind to replace *pitfall* thoughts, which generate discouragement, fatigue, and lack of motivation, with *booster* thoughts, which generate excitement, energy, and determination. As we saw in Chapter 5, your mantra is one of the most powerful thought-transforming tools you can have.

NOVELTY AND OBESITY

Novelty-seeking personality types are more likely to crave a dopamine hit and are also more likely to struggle with obesity, according to recent research. A 2015 study followed more than 600 obese women over the course of a year. Their personality traits were tested before they began a comprehensive weight-loss program. At the end of the year, a low novelty-seeking score was associated with weight loss. Low novelty seekers probably were able to resist cravings, whereas the novelty seekers couldn't resist. Naturally, novelty seeking is associated with impulsivity and the need for instant gratification. As you know, giving in to temptations can shrink the brain, and a shrunken brain only exacerbates impulsivity. Not to worry. The tools in this program will help you to tap into the power of your mind to change your brain.

Identifying Your Mantra

If you skipped Chapter 5, go back and read "Meet Your Mantra" (page 77) to find out what a mantra is and how it can help you replace pitfall thoughts with booster thoughts. If you're coping with low dopamine, your mantra is likely to express discouragement, defeat, and a sense of inadequacy. Here are some common "ravenous for dopamine" mantras:

No one truly understands me.

I'm just not good enough.

It's me versus the world.

I never really succeed.

I let people down a lot.

My life is not going the way I thought it would.

I can't finish anything.

Something has to change.

Is this all there is?

I just can't get started.

I can't do anything right.

There's got to be more to life than this.

I'm not really a good person.

I should be stronger than I am.

Something's wrong with me.

I just can't get it together.

I feel helpless.

I wish I were somewhere else.

I know it's not pleasant looking at such negative statements, but like a surgeon getting ready to cut out an unhealthy growth, we've got to identify the problem with precision before we can do anything about it. Every one of us tells ourselves a story about the world and who we are—a story that is embodied in our mantra. Our mantra tells us what we can expect, from the world and from ourselves. If we're going to change our behavior and get new results, we will get a lot further if we start by changing our mantra. But we can't *change* our mantra until we *identify* our mantra.

So what's *your* mantra? Do any of the ones on page 110 sum up your sense of yourself and the world? If so, this is your pitfall mantra. Write it down and then go right to the next section to find out how this mantra affects your weight.

If none of the statements I've supplied describes you accurately, now is the time to write down your own personal pitfall mantra. Take a few minutes and really get down the sentence or phrase that captures your core beliefs about who you are and how the world responds to you. What words do you keep hearing that make you feel discouraged, unmotivated, and inadequate? Please write them down somewhere that you can access them easily and then proceed to the next section.

How Your Mantra Affects Your Weight

As we saw in Chapter 4, your pitfall mantra has a powerful effect on your brain chemistry. Each time you repeat it to yourself—even unconsciously—your dopamine levels fall a little bit. If you feel trapped inside these thoughts, you will feel trapped inside your life, and your brain chemistry will reflect that:

> RESTRICTIVE ENVIRONMENT → ANGRY AND/OR
> DISCOURAGED THOUGHTS → LOWER DOPAMINE
> LEVELS → MORE DESPAIR AND LESS MOTIVATION TO
> CHANGE → NO ACTION, OR ONLY RECKLESS ACTION
> → MORE RESTRICTIONS IN YOUR LIFE → EVEN LOWER
> DOPAMINE LEVELS → MORE DESPAIRING THOUGHTS . . .

You can easily see how dopamine deficiency creates food addictions and weight gain. The more unmotivated and discouraged you feel, the more you reach for caffeine to perk you up while turning to high-fat foods that bring your brain some pleasure. You're ravenous for a sense of aliveness and purpose—and caffeine, fat, and perhaps risky or exciting behavior may feel like the only pleasure you can expect.

Transforming Your Mantra

Seeing how your old pitfall mantra keeps you stuck in an unsatisfying cycle—and how it contributes to weight problems—you may now be ready to choose a new, positive mantra to replace it. Here are some possible choices for a booster mantra:

When I've made a real effort to communicate with people I love, they have always been willing to help me.

There are many things I am good at, and the more I focus on my strengths, the better I feel.

I am successful in many areas of my life, and weaknesses are opportunities for growth.

There are many people who love me.

My life is not exactly how I imagined it, but there are many things that I'm proud of and still some things I'd like to achieve.

When I use successful strategies, I'm actually effective at getting things done.

There are many things that make me happy. The emptiness I'm still feeling is information that I need to change something or add things to my life.

Here I am, and I'm going to *live* this life I was given.

I'm here on this earth to find out what life wants out of me—not what I want out of life.

Choose a booster mantra from the list or create your own, writing down exactly the phrase that expresses how you would like to see yourself and the world. We'll come back to it again later, so I'd like you to have it ready. The right booster mantra can be a powerful tool in shaping your life, not to mention your body, and I want you to choose one that you feel perfectly articulates the self and the life you want.

Using the Sugar Brain Fix to Transform Your Mantra

As we saw in Chapter 5 (page 81), changing your mantra is not necessarily a simple task. No matter how often you tell yourself that you *should* feel different about yourself, the fact remains that you feel the way you feel. If you're discouraged, unmotivated, or depressed, then those are your feelings, and logic doesn't necessarily enter the picture.

However, what does change your self-concept and your mantra is *experience*. Trying out new actions and noticing the consequences allows you to re-create your life.

Check out these examples of old beliefs transformed into new ones. Can you relate to any of them?

Old Belief	New Action	New Consequence	New Belief
I'm no good.	I'm going to sign up for that Spanish class I've been thinking about.	I realized I'm quite good at learning foreign languages. I'm a smart person.	I'm good at many things.
Something has to change.	I'm going to list the three things I'm most grateful for, and I'm going to spend 10 minutes writing about the one area in my life I most want to change.	I feel happy acknowledging all that is right in my life. And when I was really honest with myself, I realized that I'm not feeling fulfilled in my work. I'm going to go to that open house at the university to see if their programs could be an option for the long term.	Life is full of opportunities to grow and change.

Taking action to create new experiences is what makes the Sugar Brain Fix effective. Going on a trip to a place you've never been, challenging yourself with puzzles and brain teasers, trying out different types of food, exploring a new hobby or a new form of exercise—all of these are dopamine-boosting actions that will allow you to see fresh possibilities, in your life and yourself. That's how to change a downward spiral into an upward spiral:

BOOSTER ACTIVITIES → POSITIVE CONSEQUENCES → BOOSTER THOUGHTS → MORE DOPAMINE → MORE EXCITEMENT, VITALITY, AND MOTIVATION → MORE ENERGY FOR MORE BOOSTER ACTIVITIES → POSITIVE CONSEQUENCES → *MORE* BOOSTER THOUGHTS → *MORE* DOPAMINE . . .

You won't necessarily be able to change everything overnight. But you can make small changes that you'll feel right away. Over time, step by step, change by change, you'll discover that you've created a new mantra—and a new life. The first step is simple: Add a few booster foods and activities to your diet and your life. After that, who knows?

Supporting Your New Mantra

As we saw in Chapter 5, I always ask my patients to create support for their new mantras by giving reasons why they're true (see page 84). Here's an example of how that might work for a dopamine-boosting mantra:

I am successful in many areas of my life . . .
because I have tried hard.
because I am talented at what I do.
because of who I am.
because when given a challenge, I rise to it.

Revitalizing Dopamine

Your goal through your 28 days of the Sugar Brain Fix is to restore your body's natural production of dopamine, which will in turn restore your ability to enjoy your life.

As a reminder, for the first two weeks, you won't deprive yourself of anything you want. You will simply add dopamine boosters: challenging activities, and foods with amino acids and plenty of vitamins and minerals. Your body will begin to make sustainable amounts of dopamine, getting you off the "buzz-crash" cycle that bad fats and excessive caffeine can create. Your cravings for bad fats will evaporate while your caffeine cravings will decrease. You'll find yourself losing weight *without even trying*, even as you still enjoy your favorite foods—but in moderation, not in excess.

Your reward will be a renewed pleasure in all aspects of your life and renewed motivation to go forward making the choices you want.

Chapter 7

FEELING POWERLESS

Starving for Everything

If a common serotonin-deficient mantra is "I don't feel safe" and a dopamine-deficient one is "I'm not good enough," the double-deficiency mantra is "Help! My life is out of control!" If you tested low in both categories, you may feel that both you and your life are out of control. You may have gone through a series of stressful events—perhaps a parent's illness, the end of a relationship, a child's crisis, or difficulties at work. You might feel that you once used to have an easy relationship with food and eating but that now, for the first time in your life, you don't. Or perhaps you always struggled with your relationship with food but now you feel it's gotten the best of you. Possibly you feel that you've always been out of control when it came to food—and perhaps to other life issues, too—and you're turning to the Sugar Brain Fix with the hope that you can finally regain control and restore your sense of personal power.

What does it mean to feel out of control? The following are some possibilities. Not all the descriptions will apply to any one person; they are a range of ways that you might feel or behave. Do you recognize yourself in any of the descriptions?

Low Serotonin Levels	Low Dopamine Levels	Low Levels of Both Serotonin and Dopamine
Attitudes: anxious, fearful, helpless, pessimistic, uncertain, unconfident	**Attitudes:** angry, depressed, despairing, fatigued, hopeless, listless, unmotivated	**Attitudes:** "at the end of your rope," confused, exhausted, frantic, "frozen," hysterical, powerless
Behaviors: obsessing and worrying constantly over relationships, money, work, or the future; avoiding decisions; feeling clingy, dependent, and needy; having difficulty falling asleep, often because of worry; frequent or continual craving of sweet, starchy food	**Behaviors:** flying off the handle at little things, often unexpectedly; feeling unable to do the simplest tasks; not being able to concentrate; frequently berating yourself for mistakes and reminding yourself of your inadequacies; shutting down thoughts and feelings in order to avoid feeling inadequate; possibly engaging in risky behaviors around gambling, drugs, sex, or physical risk; difficulty remaining asleep; frequent or continual craving of high-fat foods	**Behaviors:** alternately reaching out to people and pushing them away; crying in a way that feels out of control; forgetting things or becoming easily confused; isolating yourself; sleeping too much or too little and generally feeling helpless with regard to sleep; wanting sex far more often or far less often than usual; frequent or continual craving of both sugar and bad fats

As you can see, when both your serotonin and dopamine levels are too low, you tend to crave both sugar (indicating a serotonin deficiency) and bad fats (denoting a lack of dopamine). Because your brain chemistry is so out of whack, your cravings may be even more intense than those of the person who lacks only *one* vital chemical, as might your other responses. Where someone with a mild serotonin deficit might feel a little clingy, you burst into tears when a friend says she has to get off the phone; where someone with a moderate dopamine deficiency might be short-tempered, you find yourself erupting in rage when your spouse forgets to buy the milk. Both your internal and your external worlds may feel beyond your control, exacerbated by your frequent or continual cravings for food and your seemingly boundless appetite.

Whether this is a familiar condition or a recent development, it's profoundly dispiriting and can lead you to fall into the seven pitfall thought patterns that you'll learn more about in Part IV. You may have tried to regain control of your eating, your life, or your own responses, and if you weren't 100 percent successful, or if you couldn't maintain the control you had won, you probably felt even worse about yourself. These bad feelings depleted your stores of serotonin and dopamine still further. Then, your brain shrinks—magnifying the feelings of being powerless, overwhelmed, and out of control even more. You're trapped in another version of a downward spiral:

RECENT OR LONG-TERM LIFE STRESS OR FAMILY SITUATION → LOW LEVELS OF SEROTONIN AND DOPAMINE → FEELING POWERLESS, OVERWHELMED, AND OUT OF CONTROL → *LOWER* LEVELS OF SEROTONIN AND DOPAMINE → SHRUNKEN BRAIN → FEELING EVEN *MORE* POWERLESS, OVERWHELMED, AND OUT OF CONTROL . . .

No wonder you have cravings for brain-shrinking sugar and bad fats! If this is your situation, don't worry. The more intense, overwhelming, and out-of-control your feelings toward food have become, the more likely that a brain-chemistry imbalance and shrunken brain are involved. That's actually good news, for two reasons:

One, the problem isn't an essential one about you, your personality, or your strength of character but rather is a *fixable problem* that can be addressed with different food and lifestyle choices.

Two, I'm offering you an approach to eating that starts by add-ing brain-boosting foods and activities, *not* by taking anything away. Unlike any other diet that failed in the past, adding foods and activities rather than asking you to give something up is going to allow you the sustainable benefits of gradual detox. Any diet you've tried previously was almost bound to fail because it put you into a state of withdrawal that would be especially painful for someone who was short on both serotonin and dopamine.

The Sugar Brain Fix will ease you through the withdrawal period without your even realizing that it's happened—with con-scious tools that change the way you think and a subconscious tool by adding self-hypnosis. So let's get started. It's time to help you shift your mantra from "I'm out of control" to "I know my strengths and weaknesses, and I can make healthy decisions."

Rewriting Your Mantra

If necessary, review the sections on mantras in the previous chapters (pages 79 and 109). Then identify your current pitfall mantra. Here are some possible choices:

I can't handle anything—I'm just a mess!
I've really screwed everything up, and I'm paying for it now.
Why does everything in my life always go wrong?
No matter what I try, it's just no good—and I'm getting tired of trying.
Help! I'm out of control.

You can also write your own unique pitfall mantra, one that describes your own personal mental and emotional states.

Next, choose a new booster mantra that will support you in your efforts to restore your brain chemistry and take back your life. Here are some possible choices:

It's time I started dealing with my problems, and with some help, I'll be able to handle them.

There are things that have happened to me that weren't my fault, and now it's time to address the things that are within my control.

My life has not been perfect, but I've learned many lessons and have become stronger. With this growth, I'm ready to create the life I want to live.

I have many strengths and qualities that make me lovable. I will start by loving myself.

I won't always feel like this. These unpleasant feelings are information to create something different and better for myself.

The more things I do to feel in control of my life, the better I will begin to feel.

I'm going to be okay.

Or, once again, you can write your own specific new booster mantra—one that will help you create exactly the life you want. Take a few minutes to word it just the way you want it, and write it down.

Finally, take that new mantra and add some "because" statements to it. I'd like you to keep adding new ones as they occur to you, but take a few minutes to add at least three or four now:

I am going to be okay . . .

. . . because this time I'm going to do things differently and get the help I need.

. . . because I've felt this way in the past, and I got through it.

. . . because I'm willing to do whatever it takes to get me to the place I want to be.

. . . because I am loved, capable, and beautiful.

Now, as I've said already, I don't expect you to just jump on board with this new way of looking at the world and your life. It will take time for you to create the experiences that prove to you that your new mantra is true. I am going to help you with four exercises that can support your efforts to boost your brain chemistry.

Hindsight Is 20/20

Think back to a time when you felt really worried or angry about something that ended up being a short-lived problem. Maybe it was a nasty breakup that you thought you'd never get over. Or perhaps it was a fight with a friend, an argument at work, or a conflict with your family. Somehow or other, eventually the matter was resolved. Maybe you even thought, *What was I so worried about?* But when you were in it, the problem felt all-consuming. Impossibly heavy—and permanent.

Sit quietly for a minute and try to relive that painful time, including the memory of how nothing truly awful happened in the end. Allow yourself to absorb the truth: Those feelings were not permanent at all. Give yourself an image or a word that you associate with that memory, and next time you're sure that you'll never feel any better than you do right now, picture the image or say the word. Don't let permanence sap your brain chemistry—use this exercise to fight back.

Talk to Your Heart

Imagine that your mind and your heart each have a voice and that they are having a conversation with each other. Your heart represents the way you feel, which sometimes includes pitfall feelings. When you're hearing a voice telling you, "It's always going to be this way" or "You can't possibly get through this," that's your heart talking. It might even be saying, "Why bother?"

There's a reason the heart is giving us this message. Feelings are important information, and sometimes these despairing words are our way of telling ourselves: "Make a change! This isn't working! Do something else!"

So please don't ever ignore your heart. But do listen to what the mind is saying in response. When the emotional heart says, "I'm a terrible person and I hate myself," imagine the logical brain saying, "You're not terrible. You have good intentions in your life."

When the heart says, "Why bother? Nothing will ever change," let the logical brain reply, "But we're embarking on a 28-day journey where we'll be doing things we're never done before. Imagine at least the possibility that we might feel different in ways we can't imagine now."

Let Your Feelings Float By

Imagine that you are sitting beside a peaceful river under a tree on a beautiful day. Feel yourself actually sitting there with the grass beneath you and your legs touching each other as you sit. Now imagine that this river represents your mind and contains all the thoughts and feelings you are experiencing at the present moment. Feel the separation between yourself and the river. What's floating by may be what you are thinking and feeling, but it is not *you*. You are here on the riverbank, not there in the water.

Notice the difference between this *essence* of you, and your thoughts and feelings. Just observe them, letting each thought or feeling flow by. Look, there goes *I'm not good enough!* There goes *Nothing will ever change!* There goes *You can't lose weight, so don't even try.* There goes *No one will ever love you,* and *You fail at everything,* and *What's the point?* You might recognize all of those thoughts and feelings, but sitting here on the riverbank, can you see that they are not *you*? Don't argue, scold, or try to change them. Just watch them flow on by.

Just Do Something

I've saved the simplest exercise for last: *Just do something.* On days when you feel yourself falling into anxious or blue thought patterns and your life feels completely out of control, choose booster activities that give you a sense of *pleasure* and *productivity*. Pick a task, no matter how small—putting a book away that's been lying on your coffee table, taking the garbage out, maybe even just taking a shower. Tell yourself to do it and let yourself accomplish it. Then pick some form of pleasure—a silly movie, a five-minute walk, a phone call with a friend—and do that. If you're not sure what to do, look at the list of booster activities on pages 191 and 203 and pick one. Any one. Sometimes it's just the doing that matters.

Feeding Your Brain to Control Your Life

It's a terrible feeling to be starving for everything. It's hard not to blame yourself for your predicament, even as you feel too depressed, insecure, and confused to take steps to change it. If you are starving for serotonin and desperate for dopamine, I feel for the discomfort you are in. Your program will blend serotonin *and* dopamine boosters so that you can replenish both brain chemicals. I also want to assure you that there is a solution to your problem. Commit to the first day of the 28-day Sugar Brain Fix, and then, when that day is done, commit to the second day, and then the third, and then the fourth. Maybe it will be easier to make the commitment knowing that you don't have to give up *anything* until you're ready to do so. When the time is right, you'll take the next step—and regain control of your life.

Chapter 8

THE SECRET OF INTERMITTENT FASTING

As you know, your Sugar Brain Fix utilizes a Kediterranean diet to grow your brain while shrinking your waistline. The ketogenic-inspired element of this program includes intermittent fasting and fasted-state workouts. Without glucose from food, your body is forced to burn stored fat for fuel. When it burns fat, it releases a substance called ketone bodies. Traditional keto diets use long-term carbohydrate restriction to facilitate this process—called ketosis.

Our diet helps you grow your brain and shred belly fat with practices that encourage *mild* ketosis. With less sugar in your diet and brief fasts, blood sugar levels fall. Intermittent fasting has been shown to boost ketosis more than a standard low-calorie diet, so you'll maximize its benefits without long-term restriction.

One of the biggest myths is that skipping meals will make you eat too many calories later. A *BMJ* analysis of multiple studies of people who eat breakfast versus those who skip the meal found that the meal skippers consumed between 200 and 300 calories less per day than those who didn't. Meal skippers also tended to weigh less. As part of your Sugar Brain Fix, you'll be skipping or replacing a few meals.

This diet is also remarkably effective at reducing insulin and combating insulin resistance. When high insulin or insulin resistance is present, glucose accumulates in your blood, which can shrink your brain and expand your waistline. A study published in the *International Journal of Obesity* had two groups follow a Mediterranean diet. One group was using a Mediterranean framework but added intermittent fasting a few days per week—which is exactly what you'll be doing in your Sugar Brain Fix program. The other group kept the Mediterranean framework and simply followed a calorie-restricted diet of 1,500 calories per day. The fasting group got to eat slightly more calories overall during the six-month study. While both groups lost weight, the Mediterranean plus intermittent fasting reduced insulin levels and combated insulin resistance. The Mediterranean plus low-calorie group showed no improvement in insulin levels or insulin resistance.

In addition to its benefits on insulin, the hybrid Kediterranean template of the Sugar Brain Fix is far more sustainable over the *long term* than pure keto diets. It allows for brain-healthy foods that traditional ketogenic diets eliminate or severely restrict, like fruit and beans. Some of the amino acids, vitamins, and minerals found in fruit and beans are key for the production of serotonin and dopamine. When these feel-good chemicals are high, you feel good. When you feel good, it's easier to make healthy choices.

In this program, brief fasts are paired with workouts. By combining a short fast with exercise, you can reap the same benefits of longer fasts or strict keto. You may notice increased muscle due to the boost in growth hormone as well as energy due to an increase in adrenaline levels that comes with fasting. Since lean muscle mass increases while you're shredding fat, the number on the scale may not move that quickly. Not to worry—your weight doesn't matter as much as body composition when it comes to fixing your sugar brain. You're still becoming more healthy and fit, and you'll feel it.

What type of exercise should you be doing for fasted-state workouts? Most people do fasted-state, sustained cardio. An hour-long walk, a 45-minute jog, 30 minutes on the rowing machine, or swimming at a steady pace for 60 minutes are all great.

I also love a shorter, 30-minute burst interval training with weights and muscle training for my own fasted workouts. In general, I always say the best type of exercise is the one you like—since it's the one you'll actually do. *Adding* fasted workouts doesn't mean you should abandon your normal exercise routine on other days. In week 1, you'll add one fasted workout—but you should also be exercising nearly every day on days when you've eaten three meals.

As you know, making your waistline smaller increases the likelihood that you'll keep your brain bigger. As part of your intermittent-fasting regimen, you can either skip a meal altogether or replace it with bone or vegetable broth (check out Appendix A for broth recipes). Bone broth is the one "food" that doesn't count during a fast. Water, unsweetened coffee, and unsweetened tea are also permitted. Research shows that intermittent fasting is one of the best ways to boost a variety of hormones that help to fix sugar brain.

Intermittent fasting will also help boost serotonin levels. As you know, healthy brain chemistry is central to the Sugar Brain Fix's Kediterranean template. By increasing this soothing hormone without sugar, you'll break free from the addictive hold of food. Research has found that people practicing intermittent fasting increase serotonin levels by 33 percent after a few weeks and 43 percent over a month. Researchers have noted mood improvement, a sense of tranquility, alertness, and even euphoria after just a few days of intermittent fasting. Intermittent fasting has been shown to boost dopamine levels as well.

Thus, intermittent fasting and fasted workouts will be part of your program whether you're deficient in serotonin, dopamine, or both.

The growth hormone BDNF surges with intermittent fasting and exercise. Good news: BDNF has been shown to grow the same part of the brain that sugar shrinks: your hippocampus. The rise in the growth hormone BDNF you get by adding intermittent fasting is jaw-dropping. One study found that just a few weeks of intermittent fasting increased BDNF levels in humans by 25 percent and a whopping 47 percent after one month.

For a real triple-whammy effect, combine intermittent fasting, a fasted workout, and an infrared sauna. Research has found that subjects treated with two weeks of daily sessions in an infrared sauna lost weight and decreased fasting blood sugar when compared to a control group. Who doesn't want to burn some extra calories while relaxing? Infrared saunas are also wonderful for detoxification. See Appendix B for more information about the importance of detoxification and the infrared sauna I recommend.

Introducing Intermittent Fasting and Fasted Workouts into Your 28-Day Sugar Brain Fix

In addition to balancing your brain chemicals with the foods associated with a bigger brain, your 28-day Sugar Brain Fix adds intermittent fasting and fasted workouts to supercharge your results (this is the keto element of its Kediterranean template).

By skipping or replacing one breakfast or dinner in week 1, you'll be doing a 16-hour fast—not eating for 16 hours from dinner one night to lunch the next day. Bone or vegan broth can be used as a substitute to mimic fasting since it has little to no effect on blood sugar and insulin. This will leave you eight hours for your feeding window. Let's say your dinner on Friday night finishes at 8 P.M. If you skip breakfast and eat lunch at noon on Saturday, you have fasted for 16 hours and will then eat from noon to 8 P.M.—an eight-hour feeding window. Narrowing your feeding window is incredible for brain health and weight loss. You're also going to supercharge your results with at least one fasted-state workout. In this case, you'd exercise around 11 A.M. on Saturday morning. If you finish your workout just after noon, you can be home eating lunch by 12:30.

If you choose to skip or replace dinner instead, you're still doing a 16-hour fast. In this case, you may choose to skip Tuesday night's dinner. If your lunch Tuesday ended around 2 P.M., then your next meal would be Wednesday morning around 6 A.M. In this case, your fasted workout would occur very early Wednesday morning, around 5 A.M. Try to eat your next meal about 30 minutes after fasted-state workouts—filled with healthy, omega-3-rich protein/fat and whole fruits as your carbohydrate source to refuel, recover, and fuel muscle growth.

The meals that you will skip or replace are breakfast or dinner. That's because we're taking advantage of a time you're already fasting: when you're asleep. Thus, don't make lunch the one skipped meal. Is it better to skip breakfast or dinner? Consider your schedule and your priorities. Also, consider compliance.

Skipping or replacing dinner is more effective for weight loss, but skipping or replacing breakfast is easier. Skipping breakfast feels easier because ghrelin, your hunger hormone, is at its lowest point in the morning and highest at night. However, skipping dinner is more effective since a food eaten at night is more likely to be stored as belly fat than a food eaten in the morning. One study had overweight subjects eat exactly the same amount of calories for 12 weeks. One group ate a tiny, 200-calorie meal for breakfast. The other group ate a tiny, 200-calorie meal for dinner. The group that had a small dinner saw their waistlines shrink more while experiencing a more significant reduction in blood sugar.

Throughout your program, don't snack—although water, unsweetened coffee, or unsweetened tea with up to one tablespoon of a healthy fat like organic half-and-half is permitted. (One exception: Binge eaters who find skipping snacks increases the likelihood of a binge can add snacks between meals; see Chapter 11 on binge eating for more recommendations.)

In week 2, you'll skip or replace *two* meals and do at least *one* fasted-state workout. The most effective two meals to skip or replace this week would be two consecutive meals: a dinner and the next morning's breakfast. This choice means you're now doing one 20-hour fast this week. When two consecutive meals are skipped or replaced—dinner and the next day's breakfast— you'll still be eating two meals on each of these days, ensuring that you're consuming enough brain-boosting omega-3s, amino acids, vitamins, and minerals to support brain health.

If skipping or replacing a dinner and the next morning's breakfast feels too difficult, then skip or replace two nonconsecutive meals: one breakfast and one dinner; two breakfasts; or two dinners. By doing so, you'll be doing two 16-hour fasts this week. If you skip or replace two nonconsecutive meals, do your fasted workout just before the next meal you're going to eat. For example, do the workout just before lunch if you skipped or replaced breakfast. If you skip or replace dinner, do the workout early the next morning before the next day's breakfast.

In week 3, you'll skip or replace *three* meals and do at least *two* fasted-state workouts. Ideally, skip or replace two consecutive meals and then one additional breakfast or dinner this week. Now you're doing a 16-hour fast and a 20-hour fast in the same week. Alternatively, you could skip or replace three nonconsecutive meals: two breakfasts and one dinner; one breakfast and two dinners; three breakfasts; or three dinners (amounting to three 16-hour fasts in the same week). Fasted-state workouts will always be in the morning. If you have skipped or replaced just dinner, it will be early the following morning before breakfast. If you have skipped a breakfast, it will be in the late morning just before lunch.

In week 4, you'll skip or replace *four* meals with *two* fastedstate workouts. Skip or replace two consecutive meals, and do this twice this week. Now you're doing two 20-hour fasts in the same week. You could also do this once and then skip or replace two additional breakfasts/dinners. This would mean you're doing one 20-hour fast and two 16-hour fasts in the same week. Or, you can skip or replace four breakfasts or dinners—which would mean four 16-hour fasts this week. The timing of the fasted-state workouts will be the same as noted in week 3.

When you're done with the 28-day Sugar Brain Fix, follow the intermittent-fasting schedule and fasted-workout program that you did in week 4 for maintenance. I've found the variety of options for the intermittent fasting makes the Sugar Brain Fix program accommodating, since you can adjust the meal and workout timing based on that week's schedule.

For example, it can be hard to fast during a busy day at work. But skipping breakfast and working out on a leisurely Saturday at 11 A.M. can feel quite easy. If your nightly family dinner is something you value since you barely get to see your kids, then skip or replace breakfasts only. The variety of days when you eat normally and days with intermittent fasting keeps your body guessing. This prevents plateaus. If you drastically cut calories to the same level every day, your basal metabolic rate will dip. On the other hand, intermittent fasting *increases* your basal metabolic rate.

If skipping meals is difficult, replace them with bone or vegan broth. You can add herbs, spices, apple cider vinegar, onions, garlic, shallots, and Himalayan salt for flavor. Low-sugar vegetables like leafy greens are also permitted.

For fluids during intermittent fasting, you can have:

- water—a squeeze of lemon or lime is permitted

- mineral or sparkling water, flavored or unflavored—but not sweetened

- unsweetened coffee with up to one tablespoon of organic cream or half-and-half (milk is *not* permitted), coconut oil, or MCT oil; a pinch of cinnamon and/or stevia is permitted

- unsweetened tea—lemon and/or stevia is permitted

You can have these beverages with or between meals.

Exceptions

Children and pregnant or nursing women shouldn't use the intermittent-fasting and fasted-workout part of the Sugar Brain Fix program. If you're severely malnourished or underweight, don't use it. If you have type 1 or type 2 diabetes, have gout, gastroesophageal reflux disease (GERD), or are taking medication, consult your health-care professional before adding intermittent fasting and fasted workouts. Medication timing can often be moved, and 16- and/or 20-hour fasts are actually quite mild fasts—especially when you can replace meals with broth.

If you have a history of binge-eating disorder, I've found it's best to use broth as replacement since skipping a meal altogether can increase the likelihood of a binge. If you have a history of bulimia or anorexia, skip the intermittent fasting and fasted workouts—since food restriction is central to these serious disorders and can lead to a relapse.

Even without the intermittent-fasting and fasted-workout element, the Sugar Brain Fix program's reduction in sugars and bad fats will help you grow your brain and shrink your waistline.

See Appendix C for more details on who should not use the Sugar Brain Fix program.

WHY BONE BROTH?

Bone broth is a nutritious and delicious part of your Sugar Brain Fix. If you don't eat meat, you can substitute a vegan broth. If you do eat meat, favor bone broth over vegan broth since it contains more nutrients. Make sure it's made from bones that are grass-fed to increase the omega-3 content. When used as a meal replacement during intermittent fasting, either broth will keep blood sugar low—encouraging your body to turn to stored fat instead of glucose for fuel. Bone broth is rich in collagen and the amino acids glycine and glutamine. Amino acids are vital, because they're the building blocks of protein and muscle.

In Appendix A, you'll find delicious recipes for beef, chicken, and vegetable broth. Most canned, store-bought broths or stocks won't give you the benefits of a home-made broth that has been simmering for a day. Simmering the broth extracts health-promoting elements from the bones. If you don't have time to make your own broth, bonebroth.com has delicious, organic, and grass-fed broths that have been simmered for 18 to 24 hours. They ship their batches of fresh broth once a week. You can use the code *drmike* for 10 percent off your order.

When making your own broth, avoid bouillon cubes that contain monosodium glutamate (MSG). You can add any type of herb or spice, dried or fresh. Sea salt is wonderful. Low-sugar vegetables like onions, shallots, and greens are acceptable as well.

Now that you know the basics of sugar brain, gradual detox, intermittent fasting, and which neurotransmitter(s) you're needing, it's time to take a look at three special situations that contribute to sugar brain. They don't apply to all people, and there's a checklist in each of the three chapters to help you determine if the chapter applies to you. If it doesn't, you can skip to the following chapter. If none of the three special situations apply to you, skip directly to Part IV, where I'll walk you through the nuts and bolts of the program itself.

Before we dive in, we're going to hear another success story from my stepfather, George.

SUGAR BRAIN FIXED: GEORGE'S STORY

After I recruited my mom, I got my stepdad, George, to fix his sugar brain, too! When you can fix your sugar brain with another person, you will notice it feels easier. You have the support of a family member, and you can plan your skipped or replaced meals together. As they say, "Failure to plan is planning to fail." Together, my mom and stepdad did a lot of planning—and this set them up for success.

Like my mom, George had also been following a points-based weight-loss program with some success. Could he also supercharge his results by adding the Kediterranean template of the 28-day Sugar Brain Fix? He sure did!

BEFORE THE SUGAR BRAIN FIX

DATE: 6/7/18
WEIGHT: 182.7 lbs.
BODY FAT: 60.8 lbs. (33.3%)
LEAN MASS: 121.9 lbs. (66.7%)

AFTER THE 28-DAY SUGAR BRAIN FIX

DATE: 7/8/18
WEIGHT: 176.2 lbs.
BODY FAT: 58.7 lbs. (33.3%)
LEAN MASS: 117.5 lbs. (66.7%)

AFTER ANOTHER MONTH—FOLLOWING THE SUGAR BRAIN FIX **MAINTENANCE** PROGRAM

DATE: 8/7/18
WEIGHT: 172.6 lbs.
BODY FAT: 57.9 lbs. (33.6%)
LEAN MASS: 114.7 lbs. (66.4%)

TOTAL NUMBER OF POUNDS LOST: 10.1
TOTAL NUMBER OF POUNDS OF BODY FAT SHREDDED: 2.9

THE TAKEAWAY: Like my mom, my stepdad, George, lost more weight—simply by adding the Sugar Brain Fix program to his points-based program. He lost about 10 pounds—including about 3 pounds of fat. While his body composition percentages didn't change as much as my mom's, this is probably due to the fact that he was already exercising vigorously before he started. Also, my mom added weight-based interval training for her fasted workouts. George continued with vigorous cardio: tennis, walking, and jogging. If adding muscle is important to you, add some weight training. If simply losing fat is your goal, fasted cardio is a good choice. Or, do a little of both. Like my mom, he said that the fasting was easier than he initially thought, and he felt better.

Maintaining the Kediterranean template is easier, since he and my mom choose healthier foods *together*. Have they been perfect every week since their last Bod Pod? No. This program isn't about perfection; it's about progress. When they fell off the program for a few days or a few weeks, they just picked it back up. Have they kept the weight off (and, thus, the brain boosting) in the long term? They sure have!

Later on in this book, I'll share more success stories from people who *aren't* related to me. No matter where you are today, this program can take you even further in your journey toward better health!

Part III

SPECIAL SITUATIONS THAT FUEL SUGAR BRAIN

Chapter 9

OBSESSIVE EATING

Seeking Security

When Jennifer first walked into my office, no one would have pegged her as an insecure woman whose mantra was *I'm not safe.* She was dressed beautifully in designer clothes and had a chic Beverly Hills haircut. Recently divorced, Jennifer was frustrated by the unsatisfying relationships she kept entering and by her ongoing tug-of-war with food.

Just as no one could have seen through to Jennifer's insecurities, no one would ever have suspected her addiction to food. Yet for Jennifer, each day was one long battle. At every meal, she fought to restrict her diet to the number of calories she had determined was appropriate for the weight she wanted to maintain. In the morning, she struggled to keep from picking up snacks at the newsstand in her building's lobby. On her way home from work, she fought to prevent herself from stopping at the doughnut shop. Although Jennifer was slender and fit, she was anything but comfortable with food.

As I got to know Jennifer, I discovered she struggled with bulimia in her teens and early 20s. Now her anxieties took the form of constant diets and obsessive exercise. If she gained so much as a quarter pound, she began to panic. If she missed even a single day at the gym, she was sure that she was on her way to "looking fat and ugly." And if she ever did slip and violate her strict regime, she starved herself for days afterward, desperate to make up for what she saw as lost ground.

Jennifer's anxiety and her obsessive relationship with food were characteristic of someone who's short on serotonin. I encouraged her to consume more serotonin-boosting foods and tried to help her change her mantra. But the key for Jennifer was to tackle the addictive habits she developed. She needed to prove to herself that food was safe for her—indeed, that the world was safe.

As a cognitive-behavioral therapist I am fascinated by the interaction between behavior and attitudes. I know that the route to changing your thoughts and feelings is often to change the way you act. Actions can actually lead us to think differently, or they can reinforce the thoughts we already have. With a shrunken sugar brain, thoughts, feelings, and behavior feel difficult to change.

Jennifer experienced the world as a frightening place and, consequently, she was continually anxious. She experienced food as a powerful force that could disrupt her body and her life, and as a result, she feared that, too. My agenda was to help her prove to herself that she could give up some of her obsessive behaviors and take steps toward changing her thinking without risking her safety.

Obsessive Eating and Serotonin

People who show obsessive eating behaviors usually also have serotonin deficiency. So if you scored high on the serotonin-hungry quiz in Chapter 5, you may find that you're also trapped in obsessive behaviors. This can be one of many unique presentations of low serotonin. If you did not score high on the serotonin-hungry quiz in Chapter 5 and do not present the symptoms in the following list, feel free to skip ahead to Chapter 10.

Obsessive behaviors usually appear as an effort to regain a sense of control and safety through our actions. We're seeking security, predictability, and stability, hoping that if we control our food intake, we can control our lives.

The serotonin-boosting foods listed on page 190 in Chapter 12 will help reduce your anxiety, which should automatically help you let go of obsessive behaviors. You will also find some great serotonin-boosting meal and snack suggestions on page 246. In this chapter, I'll give you some additional support in overcoming food-related obsessions. Let's start by learning whether you *are* an obsessive eater.

Are You an Obsessive Eater?: A Checklist

Take a look at the following checklist. Check every item that applies to you.

- ☐ I need to eat the exact same thing every day.
- ☐ I feel extremely out of sorts, moody, or anxious when I can't get my usual choice of lunch/dinner.
- ☐ I like to sit and eat in the same spot every day.
- ☐ I often turn down restaurant invitations because I prefer to eat a particular food at a particular time.
- ☐ I have to have my own set of cutlery.
- ☐ I can't eat certain colored foods.
- ☐ I tell people I have an allergy when I've never been tested and there's no physical evidence I have one.
- ☐ I don't like different foods to touch on my plate.
- ☐ I have a way of eating that other people consider strange.
- ☐ I weigh my food (and have not been told to do so by a doctor).
- ☐ I get very anxious if I can't complete my exercise routine every day.
- ☐ I keep a calorie count in my head all the time.

☐ If I eat something on my "forbidden" list, I starve myself for a while or double my exercise routine.

☐ When I see someone in good shape, I have to find out what they eat.

☐ I sometimes crave foods so badly I cry.

☐ I don't allow myself to eat until I've showered/finished work/cleaned the house/done my rituals.

☐ I think the key to weight loss is eating no fat or carbs whatsoever.

☐ I hide the evidence of my eating (packaging, dirty plates).

☐ I often try to push food on my friends so I feel less guilty.

☐ I have other nonfood rituals I have to perform to feel safe.

If you checked any of these statements, your eating behavior may have some obsessive qualities, and the interventions outlined in this chapter will help you to gradually let them go. If your compulsive rituals take up a significant amount of time, if you find yourself unable to make even slight changes to them, or if your obsessions are extremely anxiety-provoking, consult a health-care professional to be screened for obsessive-compulsive disorder. If you are currently suffering from anorexia or bulimia, these are potentially life-threatening disorders that need immediate professional treatment. See Appendix C, page 313, for more details.

How Do I Let Go?

The good news here is that just as you gradually learned these obsessive rituals around food, you can also gradually *unlearn* them. If you have gravitated toward obsessive patterns around food, then we look at that as information indicating that you need more stability, predictability, or peace in your life.

Luckily, the serotonin boosters listed on page 191 will help you to put the source of stability, predictability, or peace where it belongs: in your relationships, your sense of purpose in your life, and confidence in yourself. These changes will take place as you embark on your Sugar Brain Fix, and they will also make the following obsessive-busting interventions more and more achievable.

As you now know, the most effective way to create change is through changing your experience. Even if you have specific food rules, such as foods not touching each other, you already *logically* know that your health would not be in jeopardy if you did not stick to this rule. But *emotionally*, it still feels scary. The following interventions will gradually teach the emotional part of you that you are, indeed, going to be okay, even if you take a more relaxed attitude toward food.

1. Stop weighing, measuring, and calorie-counting today.

For some people, weighing and measuring can be a great way to remain aware of what they're eating. But if you tend to obsess about your food, you will probably benefit from throwing out the scales and ditching the tape measure, and you should definitely stop counting calories and measuring food.

It may seem counterintuitive to let go of those methods of control, but we're trying to switch from a world of restrictions to a universe of abundance in which you can eat what you want and have what you need. Take a leap of faith with me and begin to act as though you don't *need* to weigh, measure, and count, because everything you want is simply going to work for you.

Set yourself up for success by starting small. Begin with a low-anxiety situation, such as a dinner where you are eating by yourself. Tell yourself, *"Just for this meal,* I will not count calories." After making yourself a reasonably sized, balanced meal, throw out the boxes with the nutritional information.

Throughout your meal, I want you to have a conversation with yourself in your head. Perhaps the emotional part of you says, "I'm feeling anxious. If I don't calculate the exact amount of calories,

I'm not going to be okay." Then imagine the logical part of you replying, "That may be the way you're feeling right now, and this makes sense, as you've been engaging in this behavior for years. But logically, you know that there is nothing dangerous about not counting calories when this is a reasonable meal that has the nutritional elements you need. You're going to be okay."

Every time you do this, the emotional part of you will begin to become less anxious. Perhaps just a small amount will change, but at least you will be slightly less anxious than before. And the person teaching you this lesson is yourself, because your experience will begin to turn off that fear.

After you've mastered that first meal, do another. And then baby-step your way to gradually bigger steps, like not counting calories when you're eating with a group. If you're listening to how your body feels, and you know you're making healthy decisions about the foods you know your body needs, you'll be well on your way to managing your anxiety. The resulting lesson will be, "I am a resourceful and strong person. I'm working on this, and I'm teaching myself that I can handle what life throws at me." Allow this improvement in self-worth to help you achieve your goals in all areas of your life.

2. Change one thing about your food rituals or habits, just to prove to yourself that you can.

One of my patients learned the benefits of this involuntarily. Spencer was a successful 40-year-old lawyer who lived in a constant state of crippling anxiety. He was obsessed with the idea that he might screw up at work, or that if he left the office before 10 P.M., he wasn't working hard enough. Spencer had always struggled with his weight and got up at 5 every morning to work out. But his eating rituals were so boring to his palate and so unsatisfying that he often craved fast food and wasted a lot of time and stress with this mental struggle. If he slipped up and ate something "off menu," he made himself run five miles. He told me that once he'd gone running at 2 A.M. because he'd eaten some fries.

Every night Spencer ordered in the exact same steak salad from the same place for dinner at his desk. Then one night disaster struck, as the restaurant changed the menu. Even though he begged and pleaded and finally became furious, the restaurant's new chef wouldn't make the old salad.

"I was so upset my palms were sweating!" Spencer told me. "I couldn't get any work done! I needed my salad to feel okay. It's hard to explain, but it was the only thing I ever wanted to eat for dinner. It was perfect, and I always felt so good eating it."

Spencer had gotten used to calming himself with food. For him, eating was an island of order and security in his hectic, frenzied life. As a child, Spencer turned to sugar and carbs to help medicate a general feeling of unpredictability and chaos during his parents' divorce. Keeping rigid control over his eating helped him feel in command, but underneath the rationality he was trying to impose lurked an addiction to foods that Spencer desperately needed to help balance his brain chemistry. And having a shrunken brain can make it feel harder to create change.

First, I helped Spencer to see what emotions he was placing on that steak salad. "Knowing exactly what I'm getting" was really a sense of familiarity and stability. Spencer and I spent some time coming up with other places to put this emotional need, so we could take the need away from the food. Luckily, his serotonin boosters helped him to meet this need by calling friends, forgiving his parents, and taking a walk outside every day. These boosters all gave Spencer an overall feeling of "I'm going to be okay."

Meanwhile, Spencer had embarked upon a serious research project: calling around restaurants looking for a steak salad like his favorite. Sadly for him, he found that no one made it the way the old place did. He ended up ordering a grass-fed steak with pepper sauce and grilled vegetables on the side.

We had rehearsed the way Spencer would get through this challenge of eating a new food. I instructed Spencer to have a conversation in his head between the logical and emotional sides of himself. So when the emotional side said, "I can't eat this. This is not the way it's supposed to be!" Spencer's logical side would reply, "I know this is hard, but you know that this new meal is not going to harm you. Every bite will be easier than the last and will help you to feel one percent less anxious."

In many ways, Spencer was being his own loving parent to his own inner, tantrum-throwing child. Although it wasn't easy, this exercise helped Spencer to get through the experience. In the end, he was surprised to discover how delicious the new dish was.

"When I was eating the new meal, I realized I was really paying attention to the flavors!" Spencer told me. "It's strange, I felt really happy and proud of myself afterward. I realized I would have felt weird if people had seen me eating the same salad every night. Of course no one ever did because I had this ritual of eating it alone at my desk. But now, trying something new, I felt free. I knew then maybe I could let go a little and it wouldn't kill me—I might even enjoy it. One night I even called my colleagues and we ate dinner together. I was still at work until 10 P.M., but at least I'm taking baby steps!"

3. If rituals around food make you feel safe, create a new ritual that is not organized around food.

If you find yourself using repetitive behavior around food, transfer some of that energy to the relationships in your life. Having a ritualized date night with your significant other or a regular night out with your best friends works as a great replacement therapy.

Bethany, 31, was obsessed with juice fasts. She would eat brain-shrinking foods for an extended period of time. When her weight reached a certain number on the scale, it was a week of all juice or cabbage soup to help cleanse, which felt miserable. By contrast, the Sugar Brain Fix's intermittent-fasting schedule is both effective and easy. You want to keep your body guessing on a daily basis to prevent plateaus—not eating whatever you want for a month followed by a week of starvation.

When I asked Bethany to share her feelings about herself and what she ate, she shook her head miserably. "I'm fat," she said simply, referring to the 10–15 pounds she was constantly battling.

"And if I eat like a regular person, I'll be huge! I know I will. I need to control my eating this way, or I'll blow up."

Actually, the truth was just the opposite: Bethany was ruining her metabolism with long periods of self-starvation, encouraging her body to cling to every ounce of fat she had and every measly calorie she consumed. Then, she would go back to eating whatever she wanted. Belly fat was stored during these long periods of time as she was shrinking her brain.

Despite Bethany's protests, I took a detour away from talking about food and weight and onto emotions and relationships. In the beginning, she didn't really see how they were all related. But I asked her, "What is it you really want, Bethany?"

She told me that what she really wanted most of all was to be in a loving relationship with a man. And then I asked about how her obsessive juice fasts were helping her to manifest her most important goal. When Bethany told me that she needed to get these last 10 or 15 pounds off, I replied, "So your current mantra is: I'm fat and no one will love me like this." She smiled and acknowledged that I was spot-on.

We then looked at how her self-critical mantra affected her achievement of weight loss. Ironically, her mantra was making it harder, not easier, to lose weight. When we come from a place of judging ourselves and believing we're unlovable, that depletes our serotonin. And guess what happens when that serotonin goes down? We feel compelled to eat sugar, and we certainly don't feel like exercising.

To Bethany, losing 10–15 pounds was the precondition for being loved. In our work together, we discovered that it was actually the other way around: Feeling lovable was the precondition for losing 10–15 pounds. If serotonin boosters could help Bethany to *feel* loved, then she wouldn't need to go on juice fasts. And instead of just getting love through romantic relationships—which are largely outside of our control—we looked at the relationships that Bethany had more control over.

We examined how establishing a girls' takeout and TV night could help Bethany to not feel so alone. When she was with her girlfriends, they always gave her the sense that what she was going through wasn't all that unusual. We all struggle with self-worth from time to time. More important, Bethany realized how much love she already had in her life.

The other serotonin booster for Bethany was creating a Monday-night yoga ritual. The calming and spiritual nature of the exercise was very healing for her, while the regularity and repetitiveness of the movements reassured Bethany and made her feel secure. Of course, it helped that yoga itself is a serotonin booster. For Bethany, it was the perfect activity, and best of all, she could practice it herself at home whenever she felt anxious. When she was tempted to self-medicate with carbs and candy, she could actually do something else that was good for her while satisfying the craving for a serotonin boost.

With this support and love, Bethany gave up her ritualistic juice fasts in favor of a sustainable way of eating. She had shifted from the sprint mentality to a marathon one. Bethany ended up losing about eight pounds and keeping it off for the long term. It wasn't her "ideal" weight, but it definitely put her in the healthy category. And when Bethany was getting love from so many places in her life and realized she was worthy of love, she was perfectly happy with where she was.

Oh, and Bethany is now dating *and* eating solid foods every day. That's a win-win!

4. If you feel anxious at just the thought of not having total control of your diet, delegate responsibility to a friend who's willing to choose a new, healthy meal for you once a week.

Vivian was a 43-year-old marketing executive who struggled with her weight and with obsessive thoughts about eating. Every day she liked to bring to work her own tuna salad, made her own particular way. She sometimes thought about eating something different or going out to lunch, but somehow she got stuck and felt antsy if she didn't stick to her routine.

I suggested to her that she literally give over control of her eating to a friend—just one meal per week—but even the thought of that upset her. Later she told me that it was as though the "private time" that she spent with her food rituals was being snatched away from her.

Vivian was tired of obsessing about her food choices, though, so she finally agreed to try this suggestion. "When I let my girlfriend decide what I would eat at lunch, I felt so angry!" she told me after her first attempt. "It was ridiculous! I'd actually *asked* her to do it, so I don't know what came over me, but I was mad."

With Vivian's overwhelming success in her work life, I wasn't surprised that giving up some personal control was a struggle for her. In some ways, it was admitting she had a weakness. But to Vivian, admitting that she was a human being who needed help every now and again was therapeutic in and of itself. In fact, Vivian's girlfriend said she felt relieved. She had always perceived Vivian as perfect and sometimes was a little afraid to confide in her. Now she felt able to get even closer to her.

After a few weeks, Vivian and her girlfriend called their Wednesday lunches "hump day lunch." The first two weeks were hard, but after that, it was quite easy. She had replaced her food ritual with a fun Wednesday lunch where she and her friend would try a new restaurant, celebrate their week, and plan for their weekends. This ended up being a much more effective serotonin booster that helped Vivian to create the life she actually wanted to live. After another month, they agreed to take turns picking new restaurants for their Wednesday outings, because going to new places and eating new things was no longer anxiety-provoking for Vivian. In fact, she looked forward to it. Ironically, the very ways she had been trying to make herself feel safe had only increased her anxiety. Opening up and becoming less isolated and more flexible paradoxically made Vivian feel safer.

Part of what makes the Sugar Brain Fix so sustainable is the flexibility it allows in intermittent-fasting schedules. For someone with obsessive eating patterns, this allows the person to not need to adhere to strict schedules. Have a breakfast meeting? Great, skip dinner so you can eat with your colleague the next morning. Did the meeting get canceled? Well, then skip it, replace it with broth, or, if you want, skip or replace dinner that evening.

Another benefit of changing her eating behaviors and improving her relationships was that Vivian felt more satisfied and therefore didn't need to snack. Intermittent fasting helps you unpair the slightest twinge of hunger with running straight to the pantry. She found she didn't need the calming sugar fixes that had kept her 20 pounds overweight since she was 25. A couple of the other serotonin boosters, such as short sessions of meditation, were extra tools in her toolbox. In the end, Vivian not only gave up her obsessive ritual but also got what she was really needing in her life.

5. Shake up your food choices by flipping a coin. When it comes up heads, eat as you normally do. When it comes up tails, force yourself to make a new choice.

This works for excessive exercise plans and obsessive calorie-counting, too. For example, if you usually run five miles or hit the gym for an hour daily, take a day off when the coin lands on tails. Or work up to the day off with baby steps, such as limiting yourself to a brisk walk instead of your demanding routine. Don't know which day to fast? Or which meal you should skip today? Flip a coin.

All of these behavior-changing exercises can achieve three goals. First, you'll learn that even if you don't have total control over your food, you'll be all right. Second, you'll be forced to focus your control issues less on food and more on other sources of stability and pleasure: family, home life, work, and your own happiness. Third, varying your eating and exercise schedule regularly prevents plateaus—keep your body guessing so that it never has a chance to adjust.

Set Yourself Up for Success

Remember, the first time you do something will always be harder than the second, or third, or fourth time. As I said earlier, listen to your heart saying, "I can't do this!" while your logical mind says, "I'm just changing my routine; it won't hurt me." You can choose which voice to listen to, even though at first, your heart will be speaking much, much louder. But every time you listen to the logical voice, it gets one percent stronger.

Of course, the whole process is slow, because your emotional voice has ruled your eating for your whole life up until now. So be patient with yourself. Set yourself up to win this fight by being kind and compassionate with your emotions. They'll come around in the end!

Chapter 10

EMOTIONAL EATING

The Search for Joy

Dede was only seven pounds over her ideal weight, but those seven pounds took up virtually all of her attention. If Jennifer's serotonin-deprived behavior in Chapter 9 was obsessive eating, Dede's dopamine- and serotonin-fueled pitfall was emotional eating. While Jennifer was a prisoner of her fears, Dede was a slave to her beliefs that she was neither attractive nor lovable. "I'm not worth anything," her mantra declared—and Dede's hangdog look, her loose-fitting clothes, and her slumped shoulders shouted that message loud and clear.

As an emotional eater, Dede ate sugar and bad fats whenever she found confirmation of her negative self-concept. Of course, since she was constantly looking for that confirmation, she usually found it! Dede was so sure she was worthless that she confirmed that opinion for herself before the world could do it for her. If she met a man she might have been interested in, rather than flirt with him or pursue a relationship, she ate. If she had an opportunity for a promotion or a new job, rather than pursue the possibility, she ate. If she spent a difficult Sunday with her mother, rather than either confront her mom or find a more satisfying way to spend her weekend, she ate.

Dede exercised excessively, so she was only seven pounds past her ideal weight. She would stay on the treadmill or elliptical trainer for hours, until she had burned a certain number of calories. Not only was this unhealthy, it was inefficient. Intermittent fasting paired with fasted workouts helps you to burn fat with short workouts—no need to spend hours at the gym.

As with Jennifer, my goal with Dede was to give her situations in which she could prove to herself that her pitfall mantra was incorrect and that her core beliefs were wrong. If Dede could truly grasp the possibility that she was lovable and worthy, she would be well on her way to freeing herself from the addictive triggers that left her looking for solace in a bag of chips.

One day, the guy Dede had liked for a long time but always avoided started dating a new woman. Dede responded by eating a whole large pizza by herself. I asked her to go back and recount the moment she knew she wanted to eat. Simply the act of recognizing her trigger was helpful in getting Dede to see herself and her behavior with a new clarity. I also wanted Dede to rewrite her story, asking, "What would the ideal Dede with a booster mantra have done in that moment?'

I had Dede practice writing down all the things she felt good about in her life. Every day I asked her to add something to the list. She began reluctantly with "My job is okay," but by day 10 she was writing about her love of fashion and how happy she was to have her best girlfriend in her life.

During the third week, Dede's mom spent all afternoon with Dede complaining about her problems. In the past Dede would have left her mom's house feeling both drained and somehow guilty for her very existence. Normally by the time she neared home, she'd know she needed ice cream and she'd stop at the store for a pint of chocolate chip and a can of whipped cream for topping. But this time, Dede gave her mom a few minutes of encouragement and compassionate listening, but not so much that Dede felt drained. Then she got up and said it was time she got home. As she walked to her car, she felt a little guilty. But she felt okay—not great, but fine—and she didn't need the ice cream.

The following week, when Dede's mom started in on her complaining, she also criticized Dede for not listening to her problems. But this time Dede had a new answer for her mom.

"I love you, Mom," she said. "But I think we both need to have some fun together. Sometimes I just feel so overwhelmed at the end of a long workday. It has nothing to do with not *wanting* to listen. It's just that sometimes, I *can't*."

Dede then pulled a DVD out of her bag—a funny romantic comedy with an actor they both liked—and suggested that they sit down together to watch it. Her mom was surprisingly upbeat afterward, and Dede knew she'd taken a big step toward letting go of emotional eating.

Doing something that gives you a sense of pleasure like watching a movie can be a simple yet effective strategy for eating more responsibly. Dede had also tested her ability to leave herself out of her mom's anxious style of thinking, and she had discovered that nothing awful had happened.

Six weeks later, Dede told me she'd met a man. There was a new guy working in her building. Dede thought he was cute, but she never thought he'd be attracted to her. She hadn't felt comfortable being flirtatious, but she had managed to look him in the eye and smile.

Dede continued to work on standing up for herself, feeling like a worthwhile person, and not suppressing her emotions while she ate her booster foods and did the booster activities I'd recommended in her Sugar Brain Fix. She started every morning with 20 minutes of learning French with an online program and opened a savings account for her dream trip to Paris. Dede needed these booster activities to remind herself that her life was full of experiences to look forward to—experiences that she could choose to create. When she chose to cook booster foods at home instead of medicating her feelings with expensive takeout, she put the $5 she had saved into her Paris fund. She wasn't focusing on what she was taking away but on what she was choosing to add.

As she reprogrammed her behavior, Dede began to notice that she didn't feel those urges to automatically eat whenever she experienced a nasty moment or a low feeling. Of course, eating foods that grow your brain make you less prone to the impulsivity and the blues that are associated with sugar brain. In fact, she felt those lows less and less often. She became friendly with the man in her office, and he asked her out for a drink.

One day she noticed four of the extra seven pounds she had carried around for years were gone. And they stayed gone. But most important, Dede's state of mind was improved. Her emotional eating habit was broken, and she was able to let go and enjoy herself.

Emotional Eating and the Brain

Sometimes I think that we've all been trained to eat in response to emotions. Commercials show people smiling and having a great time consuming some sugary doughnuts, a packaged bag of chips, or a can of soda. These images speak to your subconscious. Self-hypnosis can help to undo these unhealthy associations and plant healthy ones. Of course, many of us were taught to associate life's happiest moments with food, such as the cake on your birthday. The hippocampus and amygdala retrieve emotionally charged memories, which lead to triggers. The shrunken brain makes it feel harder to create new patterns, so you eat more and more often.

Certainly, there's nothing wrong with occasionally celebrating or comforting yourself with food. But I want your choices to be conscious and deliberate ones. Some treats, like the occasional piece of birthday cake, can continue to be celebratory parts of your life. But if you need something to make you feel better every day, then I want you to look to a serotonin- or dopamine-boosting activity. A concrete action will help you tackle the root cause of your emotional eating by getting the peace or excitement you're really hungry for.

Some of the strategies at the end of this chapter—whether you're low on serotonin, dopamine, or both—are especially helpful if you struggle with emotional eating. But let's start by finding out whether emotional eating is an issue in your life.

Are You an Emotional Eater?: A Checklist

Take a look at the following checklist. Check every item that applies to you.

- ☐ I have always felt guilty about eating.
- ☐ When I was little, I ate more than the other kids.
- ☐ I have at least one friend who makes me feel bad, but I can't seem to let him or her go.
- ☐ I had a difficult relationship with my family.
- ☐ I'm often lonely.
- ☐ When I eat, I'm not truly satisfied, even when I eat a lot.
- ☐ I eat just to have something to do.
- ☐ I always like to eat something when I get home, because it's comforting.
- ☐ I eat when other people eat, even if I'm not hungry.
- ☐ I feel powerless around food.
- ☐ I quite often feel very down on myself.
- ☐ I get very upset when I can't eat my favorite food.
- ☐ My caretaker(s) would frequently give me food as a reward when I was small.
- ☐ I feel quite disconnected from my body sometimes.
- ☐ I berate myself in front of the mirror a lot.

☐ My desire to eat comes from above-the-neck emotional hunger, rather than below-the-neck physical hunger.

☐ I have gone through phases of trying to limit my eating, but sometimes I eat a whole box of food without really noticing.

☐ I often eat in front of the TV.

☐ I've noticed I'll crave sugar and bad fats when something unpleasant has happened.

☐ I want to eat at weird times of the day and sometimes wake in the night wanting to snack.

☐ I sometimes feel overwhelmingly sad before eating.

☐ Other people push me around, and I always treat myself with food afterward.

☐ I find it almost impossible to stand up for myself, and I eat to cover how that makes me feel.

☐ When I say no, I feel guilty—and I often eat to comfort myself.

If you checked one or more of these statements, you have some form of emotional eating behavior, which probably indicates either low serotonin, low dopamine, or, in many cases, *both*. The interventions outlined in this chapter will help you to gradually let them go.

Don't despair—you can break the cycle and change not only the way you feel about yourself but also the way you react to difficult, unpleasant, or overwhelming feelings. If you are unable to make even slight changes or are experiencing any major symptoms of depression, anxiety, or other mood disorders, see a health-care professional to be screened and treated.

Emotional Eating and Your Brain Chemistry

If you're dopamine deprived, you tend to feel as though life has lost its luster. You might feel empty and down or overwhelmed and drained. You might crave drama and thrills to lift you out of your slump, or you might just long for something pleasurable and fun to relieve the daily stress.

If you're serotonin starved, you might feel anxious and on edge, worried about your work, relationships, or personal life simply slipping out of control. Or you might feel unconfident and pessimistic, fearful that nothing will work out for you, or perhaps even certain that it won't.

If you're short on both types of brain chemicals, you may simply feel that life has gotten away from you. You might believe that you don't have the energy or clarity to make changes or pursue your goals—that it's all you can do just to get through the day.

In all of these cases, you may well engage in what I call emotional eating: eating in response not to physical hunger or nutritional need but rather as the result of emotional challenges. By overwhelming the pleasure centers of hunger, you no longer eat based on physical cues of hunger from the hypothalamus. A shrunken brain makes unhealthy eating feel hard to change.

As we have seen, emotional challenges are physical, too. When you feel depressed, overwhelmed, stressed, sad, blocked, or disregarded, your brain chemistry responds accordingly. Your stores of dopamine and serotonin are depleted, and you need more biochemical support for the challenges you're facing, making your desire to eat sugar and bad fats feel as strong as the hunger you feel after hours of heavy physical labor.

The solution, as we have seen throughout this book, is to feed your brain with the foods and activities it needs to manufacture a nice, steady supply of the serotonin and dopamine on which it relies. Add intermittent fasting and fasted workouts to boost the growth hormone BDNF to grow the brain while shredding belly fat. Then you'll always feel "fed" and full, and you won't need quick fixes. Meanwhile, I can offer you some specific suggestions for rewriting your emotional eating patterns into healthier and more satisfying rhythms.

How Do I Start Feeling Full?

Luckily, if you load your life with the serotonin- and dopamine-boosting foods and activities I suggest in Chapters 12 and 13, a lot of your emotional eating will disappear on its own. Your brain chemicals will be replenished in a healthy, stable way, and you simply won't feel the pull of emotional eating as you did before.

The other way to start feeling full is to focus on specific actions that will make you feel positive and satisfied about your life. Since the most effective way to create change is through changing your experience, anything you do to improve your life will alter the way you feel about food. The more important other experiences become, the less important eating will seem—and that process will happen naturally, and without effort. If you'd like to let go of some of your emotional eating patterns, give one of the following suggestions a try.

1. You are good enough.

Do one thing that will make you feel "good enough" today. You might push yourself to just smile or say hello to someone in the elevator, make a $5 donation to an animal rescue group or pediatric cancer foundation, or call a friend who always seems to "get" you. Connecting to your ability to make a difference reminds you how many worthy and lovable qualities you have. There's also nothing wrong with trying to make yourself feel as good as possible on the outside when you feel lousy on the inside. When I feel down or have been mourning a loss, those are some of the moments when I decide to put on my favorite shirt, shave, and comb my hair.

2. Sign up for your future.

Take a positive step toward a goal by trying something new. If you've always wanted to learn to paint, sign up for classes. If you've secretly always yearned to be a dancer but thought you weren't graceful enough, find a beginner's class and enroll today. If you have a dream vacation, open a savings account. Notice how you're filling your life with two more of the seven booster qualities: productivity and purpose. You can find more suggestions for booster qualities in Chapter 14.

3. Detach from situations that drain you.

In my experience, people who are prone to emotional eating are often the caretakers in a relationship. If that sounds like you, try this: Next time you're with people who are talking about their problems, see what happens if you don't do anything. Try to tolerate their unhappiness without trying to fix it. This should also help you build tolerance against your own moods the next time you feel unhappy, and so your unhappiness will be less likely to translate into hunger. You don't have to fix anything.

4. Invite and write some love letters.

Ask the five people closest to you in the world to e-mail you the three things they like best about you. Tell them you're on a journey to transform negative self-talk into self-love. Notice your reactions when you read the e-mails. Do you feel like arguing with them? Pointing out your flaws? Wondering why they picked those good qualities and not others of which you are prouder or that you wish you had? Take some time to notice how many of your thoughts had to do with fears of people mocking you or dismissing you rather than expressing their appreciation. Then write back at least a brief love note to each participant, expressing your gratitude for the joy they bring into your life.

5. Meditate.

Engage in mindful meditation, where you practice simply observing your feelings rather than trying to respond to them. Take five minutes a day to just sit quietly and practice watching your thoughts come and go. You can build up to 30 minutes or longer with practice, but start slowly, as sometimes it can be tough to quiet your thoughts. Some people find it helpful to choose a word or phrase they enjoy and repeat it in time with their deep breathing. I always tell my patients, "If you don't take your feelings so personally, your feelings won't take you so personally!" That extra distance from your feelings might give you a little more space to start making other decisions around food.

6. Take a thoughtful walk.

Grab the dog, call a friend, or simply take a brisk walk around the block *before* you give in to your emotional eating urge. As you walk, really feel your body. Feel your legs move and notice the tingle in your feet as they hit the road. Feel your breathing and notice how the air smells. Listen to the sound of the birds or passing cars. Pay attention to the way the light hits the trees. Say hello to anyone you pass, smiling and looking them in the eye. Pick up your feet, don't shuffle, and, if you can, adjust your posture so you're standing tall as you walk. Move as though you feel good about yourself, even if you don't. Studies show that with practice, behaving as though you feel good actually *makes* you feel good. You've lifted your mood with the booster attributes of power, pride, and pleasure, which might replenish your brain chemistry instead of the food you would normally choose.

7. Distract yourself.

Most cravings last about two minutes and are satisfied by about four bites. So if you can just distract yourself for a little while, you might simply forget about being hungry. Try the booster activities on pages 191 and 203, or do one of the items on the following list:

- Brush your teeth.
- Clean your kitchen counters.
- Chew some sugar-free gum.
- Floss.

- Go online and read a blog post.
- Listen to an uplifting song, and if you can, dance to it.
- Plan a family day out.
- Put on a teeth-whitening strip.
- Take a shower.
- Unload the dishwasher.
- Write a quick friendly e-mail to someone you like.

8. Make a gratitude list.

Sit down and write a list beginning with the words "I am grateful because . . ." and then think about everything that is good in your life, no matter how small. It could be anything from "I have nice hair" to "I have a great relationship with my son" to "The weather was good today." As soon as you start looking for things to feel good about, you'll be surprised how many there are. Keep the list with you and add to it whenever you feel moved to do so. Read it whenever you feel like emotionally eating and see if you can feel even a little bit of serotonin or dopamine flooding back into your brain.

9. Give yourself a break.

We often think that the best way to move forward is to criticize ourselves for anything we do wrong, hoping to keep ourselves in line and avoid the same mistakes in the future. In fact, the best way to improve is exactly the opposite: to forgive ourselves for our mistakes and let them go as quickly as possible, and to focus on what we've done right. Several studies in sports psychology have found that if an athlete makes a mistake, self-talk such as "I'm trying so hard!" and "I don't give up, good for me!" is far more useful than "I just dropped the ball—what an idiot," or "I shouldn't have done that."

I suggest the same approach to you: Whatever your results with regard to emotional eating, focus on what you've done right, even if it seems like merely a tiny piece of the big picture. Self-criticism only lowers your serotonin levels, leaving you feeling low and then making you want to emotionally eat again.

10. Be mindful.

One of the greatest gifts we can give ourselves—in the midst of any grief, fear, anxiety, or depression—is to just be here now. The present moment is the only place where we can be fully at peace, the place where everything just *is* and we don't have to imagine what might be or will be, where we don't have to fret about what we've just done or failed to do. In the present, we just *are*. If you can be mindful and eat mindfully—really tasting and savoring your food—you can indulge in the pleasure of the food so that even if eating is an emotional choice, you can satisfy the craving in a few bites rather than continuing past the point where you don't feel any pleasure in it.

Here's an exercise in mindfulness that might give you some practice in mindful eating:

Take a grape, or a similar small food, such as a slice of fruit or a nut. Now pretend that you are an alien and have never encountered this object before. At first, you're not even quite sure it's a food. Touch it. Smell it. Then, taste it. Sit quietly with your eyes closed and do not chew. Simply let the food sit in your mouth. Notice any flavors or smells with your whole mouth. Really experience the food's smooth, elastic skin or the crunch of the apple. Feel the food's texture on your tongue. Roll it around in your mouth and taste the flavors as it warms up. Keeping your eyes closed, really notice the changes in texture and flavor as you slowly start to chew. Chew the food at least 50 times—more, if you can—to notice how it feels to keep food in your mouth rather than swallowing it instantly. When you do swallow, feel the food travel down your throat and enter your stomach. Sit quietly for a moment to absorb the sensations fully. Then, imagine what would change it you ate all foods more mindfully.

Putting Your Emotions in Perspective

I want my patients to get in touch with their feelings—to celebrate and honor their emotions. But I also want them to keep their feelings in perspective, rather than letting them run their lives.

I want the same thing for you. I want you to respect your feelings, but I want you also to listen to your rational side, the one that helps you have a different dialogue within your mind and heart. If you give yourself the booster attributes, foods, and activities that feed your brain chemistry and nourish your life, your feelings will get the support they need, and you'll be able to let go of emotional eating almost without trying. Both your weight and your emotions will benefit. You'll grow your brain as your waistline shrinks. The more your brain grows, the easier it is to sustain these healthy choices.

Chapter 11

BINGE EATING

Regaining Control

When I met my patient Jenna at age 28, she was in tough shape. With dark circles under her eyes and the habit of constantly picking at her fingernails, she was clearly so anxious and in so much emotional pain that she was barely functioning.

"I've always taken things very personally," she admitted. Jenna had a great memory and felt everything deeply. Every experience was almost painfully intense for her.

Jenna had come to me following a bad breakup. Unable to move on from the feelings of rejection, she had slipped back into her teenage habit of binge eating and now, locked in a cycle of strict diets and all-out gorging sessions, she had a hard time keeping self-hatred at bay.

Binge eaters may be either serotonin deficient or dopamine deprived, but most of the time they are both. Most binges are made up of both sugar and bad fats, as evidenced by Jenna's binges of pizza, ice cream, candy, crackers, fries, and soda.

The key to putting an end to compulsive eating is to create a feeling of abundance (no food is forbidden) and a sense of order (eating comes at regularly scheduled times, hungry or not). If you are a binge eater, don't skip meals as part of the intermittent-fasting regimen. Replace them with broth instead.

If you're a binge eater, you are by definition in the grip of intense spikes and crashes of various brain chemicals, as well as blood sugar, and you've long ago lost touch with genuine hunger. You might also feel a great deal of shame about your out-of-control eating. Encouraging you to eat three meals every day—whether or not you have also binged—is the first step in helping you regain control.

To increase the amount of time your body has to turn to stored fat for fuel, I generally don't recommend snacking. However, binge eaters are the exception. If you need to snack between meals, do so. For binge eaters, this can decrease the likelihood of a binge. Make your snacks foods that are high in fat first and protein second. Save your fruit servings for mealtimes. For example, avocado, nuts, or organic string cheese would be ideal snacks. Or, try veggies with hummus.

Jenna began her 28-day plan with both serotonin- and dopamine-boosting foods and activities, and with my encouragement for her to plan out all her meals in advance. That way, she could feel more control over her eating and would be less likely to slip into a binge.

But the first time Jenna came to see me after beginning the program, she was sobbing.

"I was sure I'd get fat if I ate normally," she told me. "So I cut out the two snacks and skipped breakfast. Then I just felt like I couldn't do it anymore, so I ate."

"And what did you eat?" I asked.

"Bread. A whole loaf," she cried. "Then I punished myself for the next 12 hours by not eating anything, and that led to an even worse binge! I'll always be like this. It's just the way I'm made! I'm weak and oversensitive. Why can't I just get over things like other people? Why don't I have any self-control?"

Gently I explained to her that her problem was not her sensitivity. Rather, it was that she hadn't learned to celebrate and be proud of who she really was. Instead, she constantly berated herself, bringing her mood down lower than ever. What she needed was a steady stream of serotonin and dopamine boosters and some cognitive behavioral tools to help her make the decisions she truly chose and then to stick to them. Binge eaters shouldn't skip meals. When using intermittent fasting, replace meals with broth.

"You are not allowed to feel bad about relapsing," I told her firmly. "And I also don't want you skipping any meals or snacks, whether you binge or not. If you relapse again, you will. If you relapse 20 times, you will. One day you won't. And meanwhile, you'll keep eating normally. Now move on to planning tonight's meal. Tomorrow is another day, and you can take this a day at a time."

Together we worked on changing Jenna's low opinion of herself. I had her meditating every morning for 5–10 minutes as she practiced clearing her mind of thoughts and just observing her feelings as if from a distance. She also worked on changing her inner mantra of "I'm not good enough" to "I'm worth it." (For more on mantras, go to pages 79 and 109.)

To help reset Jenna's binge eating, I also made sure she kept a journal about her feelings along with everything she ate. I also made her throw out her scales and allowed her to weigh herself only once each week, in my office. We agreed to do blind weighing so that I alone would know her weight until 28 days had passed. That's because Jenna was so obsessed about her weight that knowing it even weekly made her more anxious. Also, sometimes a person who has been starving and bingeing may see his or her weight go up before it goes down. With fasted workouts, you will likely be gaining muscle mass as you're shredding fat—so the number on the scale may not change even though your body and brain have. I didn't want Jenna to feel discouraged.

And indeed, Jenna gained two pounds at first, simply from her body's reaction to regular eating. On a constant yo-yo of all-out starving and all-out bingeing, her metabolism had become sluggish, and she wasn't burning calories efficiently. But with support from the friends and family I encouraged her to confide in, Jenna didn't lapse back into her binge-starve cycle. If you notice that replacing meals with broth leads to a binge, then don't use intermittent fasting at all; the other components of the Sugar Brain Fix are still effective without it.

During this period I also helped Jenna learn to eat in public without panicking. Her fear of food and her tendency to binge in secret had made eating in restaurants and in front of people a difficult experience. First she went to a cozy little café for lunch. She had a serotonin- and dopamine-boosting Niçoise salad rich in omega-3s, amino acids, and vitamins. She took a book with her to help her feel less self-conscious about sitting alone.

The next time, she went to the café with a friend who knew all about her issues. Jenna felt anxious at first and even told me later that having her friend there had made her feel as though she should eat only half of her meal. She stuck to the plan and left the restaurant satisfied—but half an hour later, she wrote in her journal that she wanted to eat a whole chocolate cake. Eating in public was one of her worst triggers. But then she looked at her meal plan and knew she could have a snack in two hours' time if she needed it. Jenna relaxed, and the chocolate cake remained on the store shelf.

After three weeks her body was stabilizing. She felt hungry at mealtimes and was then hugely relieved to find that she was allowed to eat a meal without guilt. Later in the evenings she felt that she didn't need to binge. She was satisfied. Leaving the daily guilt cycle behind, she began to feel better about herself and she saw herself as less isolated and more like other "normal" people.

By now, Jenna could eat in a restaurant without panicking. In fact, she went to a work lunch, and instead of avoiding food in front of her intimidating clients and then gorging on fries afterward, she ate a healthy lunch and stuck to her plan.

Of course the triggers were still in Jenna's life. Her exboyfriend still haunted her. To Jenna, the way her relationship had ended confirmed the fear that she wasn't good enough. But now, with the self-esteem-boosting work she had done, Jenna saw that she had options. She could go on a dinner date, and she could let a man fully into her life. She no longer had anything to hide. Knowing that she was no longer trapped in her secret binge-eating behavior gave Jenna the freedom to enjoy herself, while eating regular healthy meals reset Jenna's behavior, boosted her brain chemistry, and grew her brain. Her increased serotonin and dopamine levels ensured that her mood stayed on an even keel.

Jenna lost 5 pounds over the 28 days of her program, and she has been slowly and steadily losing the next 15 pounds toward her goal weight of 145 pounds. What was most surprising to Jenna was that she actually lost weight over the course of 28 days, even though she was not allowed to skip any meals! Jenna had spent most of her life starving herself for half the week or more. It seemed ironic to her that by eating more normally, she *lost* weight. But this is exactly what happens.

Why Am I Like This?

Binge eaters generally experience the world as a very intense place. They are often creative, deeply sensitive, intuitive types who are likely to have strong emotional reactions. These individuals often feel "different" or isolated due to their sensitivity and are prone to low feelings as a result. They might self-medicate with drugs, alcohol, or food, or simply isolate themselves from situations that they fear will provoke bad feelings. That's partly because someone who tries to self-medicate with a substance has never fully learned how to self-soothe. Where someone else might say, "You can handle this" or "You're better than that," the low-serotonin-and-dopamine binge eater doesn't have the brain chemical support or the childhood training to get through a challenging experience without a self-medicating binge. The more binges shrink the brain, the more blue, stuck, impulsive, and foggy they feel.

Of course, the sensitivity that leads to these intense feelings also leads to artistic, political, and spiritual insight. Great artists, poets, musicians, and writers all share this trait, as do many spiritual leaders and humanitarians. Managing the low points of this sensitivity is important, however, and part of that is seeking a supportive plan that works for you. The Sugar Brain Fix, with its support for your brain chemistry and its booster activities, can help you find both the chemical and personal support you need.

Foods with amino acids, vitamins, and minerals will help you manufacture steady supplies of serotonin and dopamine. This should ease the need to binge. In this chapter, I'll also provide you with a range of approaches that can assist you in making calmer and less impulsive choices. The first step is to find out what role bingeing has in your eating habits.

Am I a Binge Eater?: A Checklist

Take a look at the following checklist. Check every item that applies to you.

- ☐ I feel guilty, depressed, or ashamed after eating.
- ☐ I eat to the point of feeling uncomfortably full or even of being in pain.
- ☐ I eat what most people would consider a very large amount of food in a short amount of time.
- ☐ I eat a large amount of food when I'm not physically hungry.
- ☐ I avoid social situations where food is present.
- ☐ When I eat, I'm often not truly satisfied, even when I eat a lot.
- ☐ I attribute nearly all my success or failure to my weight.
- ☐ I feel powerless around food.
- ☐ I quite often feel very down on myself.
- ☐ I feel a lack of control when I begin eating.
- ☐ I enter a trancelike state when I begin eating.

☐ I feel quite disconnected from my body sometimes.

☐ I berate myself in front of the mirror a lot.

☐ After a binge, I will compensate by restricting the amount of food I will eat at the next meal or during the next day.

☐ I often eat in front of the TV.

☐ I eat very rapidly.

☐ I crave sugar and bad fats when something unpleasant has happened.

☐ Most of my eating occurs late at night.

☐ I sometimes feel overwhelmingly sad before eating.

☐ My binges occur in private because I'm embarrassed about how much I eat.

☐ I have ritual foods that I will obtain to binge on.

☐ I feel anxious once I begin thinking about obtaining my foods and my upcoming binge, but I feel that I can't do anything to stop it.

☐ I pretend that the food I buy is not all for me in some way, such as going to different drive-through restaurants or telling the takeout people that I'll need more than one set of utensils.

☐ I hoard foods—especially foods with sugar and bad fats.

If you checked any of these statements, you may have difficulty with binge eating, which probably indicates either low serotonin, low dopamine, or, in many cases, *both*. The interventions outlined in this chapter will help you to gradually let go of these difficulties. If your binge eating is excessive, and if you find yourself unable to make even slight changes, consult a health-care professional for screening and treatment of binge eating disorder. If you are currently suffering from anorexia or bulimia, be aware that these are potentially life-threatening disorders that need professional treatment.

RIDE THE WAVE

Think of your hunger as an overpowering wave that you want to learn to ride. When you introduce regular, planned eating, it's as though you're learning to surf and learning how to paddle. When you skip meals, it's as though you're helplessly hanging out on your board in the ocean. When the wave comes, you're not paddling, so it knocks you off your board and you're swept into the proverbial undertow of binge eating. Unlike intermittent-fasting strategies where a short fast is followed by a normal-size meal, this undertow makes you consume the equivalent of three or four meals in one sitting.

By contrast, people who eat regular meals are always paddling, so when their waves come, they surf them. Their waves are manageable, while for you, skipping meals leaves you open to drowning.

That's why I don't want you to think of yourself as "on a diet" or to allow yourself to feel deprived in any way. You'll be vulnerable to binges and will let the wave ride you instead of you riding it.

What's Your Trigger?

In a study on binge eating, researchers discovered 11 main triggers:

1. Tension—91 percent
2. Eating something—84 percent
3. Being alone—78 percent
4. Craving specific foods—78 percent
5. Thinking about food—75 percent
6. Going home—72 percent
7. Feeling bored and lonely—59 percent

8. Feeling hungry—44 percent

9. Drinking alcohol—44 percent

10. Going out with someone who might be a romantic partner—25 percent

11. Going to a party—22 percent

Think about your own triggers and write them down. It's important to be mindful of when you're most vulnerable, and it will also allow you to combat your triggers with booster activities. When you fill your life with things that promote healthy relationships while decreasing isolation and loneliness, you'll find that your triggers won't be as powerful. And, of course, booster foods will help you to stabilize your feel-good chemicals and grow the brain—decreasing the urges to binge.

COMPULSIVE EATERS COME IN ALL SHAPES AND SIZES

Weight and binge eating are not really related. Most binge eaters are not overweight, and most obese people—some 90 to 95 percent—don't binge.

Be Kind to Yourself

If you binge, you may also have trouble asserting yourself. You might feel that you are never good enough. You may have standards that are quite high and that you believe you do not meet. And you might isolate yourself from people or situations in which you would find yourself feeling as though you had fallen short or even failed.

That's why I'd like you to be as kind to yourself as possible, adding booster activities and foods and giving yourself all the support you can manage. Treat your state of mind as you would an innocent child. Recognize that your impulses are triggered by feeling low, and that when you're mean to yourself, you feel lower.

I also want to encourage you to set achievable goals. Don't focus on the big picture of what you'd like to do someday. Pick something to accomplish this week. This is important both for weight-loss goals and for other tasks. Small, steady, measurable gains will make you feel better about yourself, your life, and your ability to succeed. Set yourself up for success by choosing this approach.

Breaking the Cycle of Fear and Fat

Often, if you binge, you're actually scared of food, because you think that the food itself will cause you to binge. You find yourself feeling paralyzed, thinking of food at every turn, terrified of the feelings that you might experience just from being around food.

The solution? An approach known as graded exposure therapy. With this method, you can go at your own pace and take very small steps toward freedom. I used this approach with Jenna when I had her eat out alone, then with a friend. Try the following exercise yourself to see how this technique might be helpful to you.

Exercise: Face Your Fear

- Eat in front of someone at home (preferably this person is supportive and aware of your struggle).

- Eat in a restaurant or café that you find comfortable and unintimidating.

- Eat again in that same restaurant, but this time bring a good friend you feel you can trust and be relaxed with.

- Go to the same place (or another you are equally comfortable with) and eat with people you're unsure of or who give you anxiety, such as a colleague or family member.

- Choose a new, scary, and intimidating restaurant and eat with a person or group that makes you anxious or tense, such as attractive friends of friends, colleagues, or a difficult family member.

Repeat these steps until you can do each one without terrible anxiety. If a binge is triggered, accept that as part of the process and go through the steps again. Your goal is to feel somewhat less bad and somewhat less frantic to escape. Moving away from avoidance one baby step at a time will help you to conquer your fear without being overwhelmed. Give yourself credit for any effort you make and for even the smallest improvement.

Rules to Live by for Binge Eaters

- **Have a plan.** Binge eaters need to stick to a plan of three meals every day—with the option of having snacks between meals if needed. Map out what you will eat the next day and shop and prepare for this in advance. I advise investing in lunch bags or boxes to take your food to work. Think ahead. If you're unprepared, you're more likely to fall into a binge.

- **Never skip meals.** Punishing yourself by skipping a meal is the cornerstone of binge eating. If incorporating intermittent fasting, use broth as your meal. If you still feel urges to binge with this strategy, don't use intermittent fasting at all. First come the low feelings of guilt, then the self-punishment and even lower feelings, then finally the real hunger hits you and you start to crave a binge.

- **Enjoy food.** You don't have to eat food that's bland or unenjoyable. Remember, you are not allowed to beat yourself up or feel deprived on this plan. Find booster foods that you'll enjoy. When planning your meals, think about the flavors you really like. You can find some great simple recipes on pages 277–308 so you can create an entire meal out of boosters. You can even boost your brain chemistry with pancakes!

- **Never say never.** If you say, "I'm never going to eat this food," it increases the possibility of a binge. Don't encourage impulse eating by keeping your trigger foods at home, but at the same time, never say never to them or they'll be calling your name from the store. Tell yourself, "I can have that later," or work a small amount of something you crave into tomorrow's meal plan.

- **Keep a journal.** Writing down what you eat helps keep you accountable to yourself and whomever you choose to share your Sugar Brain Fix journey with. Journaling is a key part of this program, so go to the journal section on page 240 and make sure you are keeping a full and honest track of your food.

- **Weigh yourself only once a week.** Obsessing over the scale will expose you to emotional ups and downs that can trigger a binge. Everyone's weight varies a little throughout the day, so don't pay too much attention to each weekly weight reading. It's better to consider your weight over a period of four weeks or, better yet, a year.

- **Find a friend.** One of the most common characteristics of binge eaters is secret eating. Eat with others and enjoy their company!

- **No distractions.** Don't eat in front of the TV, in the car, or while working. Be present when you're eating rather than distracted by something else. Bringing this awareness to your eating will also teach you to savor your food and eat more slowly. It helps to promote the opposite of the trancelike state that is one of the characteristics of binge eating.

- **Clear your cupboards.** Decrease pitfalls and increase availability of booster foods in your home. If packaged foods are opened, it's too easy to say to yourself, "Oh well, it's open now, I have to finish it." Donate your packaged pitfalls to a church or homeless shelter and stock your shelves with healthy options.

- **Lunch money.** If you worry about eating too much while out of the house, restrict how much money you carry and leave the credit card at home. If your lunch at work is $10, take just $10 with you.

- **Hands off.** Don't taste when cooking. You'll be tempted into eating everything you've made. Treat cooking your meal like a job. You're creating a healthy dinner for you or your family, and you must complete the task without tasting it. If you really need an opinion, ask a friend or a family member to taste the food.

- **Chew gum.** Eating is an anxiety reliever, like smoking. So chew sugar-free gum to give your mouth something to do. There are several brands on the market without artificial sweeteners, like PUR Company's gum.

- **Go public.** If you love a particular food and have avoided it because you're afraid it might trigger a binge, challenge this belief by joining some friends and consuming one serving of the forbidden food. Forcing yourself to enjoy a food publicly that you normally see as forbidden and secret can go a long way toward breaking its obsessive hold on you.

Freeing Yourself from Bingeing

The principles of the Sugar Brain Fix can help free you from a problematic relationship to food and from yo-yo dieting. If you are still experiencing binge eating after completing the Sugar Brain Fix, don't berate yourself. Instead, take what you have learned and put those tools in your toolbox. Look at the continued bingeing as feedback that you may need to add another tool in the form of professional help.

Where Do I Go from Here?

By now you have learned how to free yourself from some of the most common and addictive patterns people develop around eating. These tools will help you overhaul your diet, which we're going to discuss in depth in the next section. Over the course of the next 28 days you will finally be freeing yourself from the addiction to foods that shrink your brain and expand your waistline.

SUGAR BRAIN FIXED: BRIANNE'S STORY

Brianne is an athlete in her early 30s. She does rugby, Cross-Fit, and extreme competitive competitions like Spartan Races. Brianne has always been one of those naturally fit and athletic people. Despite her athletic prowess, Brianne needed my help.

Brianne was experiencing something we'll all face at some point: a slowing metabolism as a result of aging. In her 20s, Brianne could eat whatever she wanted and not gain a pound. Now in her 30s, Brianne noticed excess weight or stored fat took her *months* to work off—even with her intense workouts. Brianne was hoping the Sugar Brain Fix could help her shred the belly fat that she was beginning to notice.

Brianne was also dealing with high levels of stress. She was pursuing her doctorate while working. Between her job and school, Brianne was working 80 hours per week. She barely had time to eat—let alone cook healthy food.

Additionally, Brianne had just lost her grandmother. Her grandmother raised her and was the most important person in her life. Understandably, Brianne reported feeling both anxious and blue when she began the Sugar Brain Fix and had recently gained 20 pounds. Brianne hoped the serotonin boosters could help her experience a little peace and relief.

Could the Sugar Brain Fix help someone who was already in pretty good shape? Brianne's body fat was still relatively low despite her recent weight gain. Could the 28-day program help her return to her former glory and grow her brain while shrinking her waistline? Could it help an overworked, grieving young woman to feel better?

There was no Bod Pod in Brianne's area, so she did two sessions of hydrostatic weighing (also known as dunk tanks) to measure her body fat composition. Dunk tanks are nearly as accurate as Bod Pods, but there are a few drawbacks. Athletes like Brianne can have dense bones, and this can throw off dunk tanks' readings. Additionally, they're subject to error if you can't fully expel *all* of the oxygen out of your lungs while you're dunking yourself. That being said, all these tests are far more accurate than calipers or devices that you have to hold or stand on a metal plate. Dual energy X-ray absorptiometry is the most accurate of all these methods, but it can cost up to $400.

Over the 28-day program, Brianne lost 3 pounds. Today, she's 9 pounds thinner than when she started. Although her dunk tank's body composition didn't reflect it, Brianne reported she absolutely noticed an increase of muscle and shredding belly fat during the 28-day program, and she took before-and-after photos to prove it. Over the long term, she continues to be extremely successful. She has now lost a total of 9 pounds.

BEFORE THE SUGAR BRAIN FIX

DATE: 6/22/18
WEIGHT: 149.8 lbs.
BODY FAT: 34.5 lbs. (23%)
LEAN MASS: 115.3 lbs. (77%)

AFTER THE 28-DAY SUGAR BRAIN FIX

DATE: 7/23/18
WEIGHT: 146.3 lbs.
BODY FAT: 35.4 lbs. (24.2%)
LEAN MASS: 110.9 lbs. (75.8%)

TODAY

DATE: 2/16/19
WEIGHT: 141 lbs.

THE TAKEAWAY: The Sugar Brain Fix is a program that can help people who are out of shape or in great shape improve their brains . . . and bodies! I'm always happy to hear people *feel* better—especially when that someone is going through rough times. This was certainly the case for Brianne.

Here's what she had to say about her Sugar Brain Fix journey:

"Thank you! Your program completely helped me jump-start my way back to fitness. I was in a serious slump for a while there. . . . Honestly, it changed my life."

Here's what she liked most about the program:

- Of all the programs I've tried, and I've tried many, this was the easiest one to stick to. And if I fell off, I was able to get right back on. With other programs, once I fell off, I was off.

- It forced me to find time to enjoy life again in little way (taking my dog for a walk, meditating, taking a bath, going for a bike ride).

- The cravings were minimal. I attribute this to the way in which the program slowly weans you off the bad stuff and gets your body wanting the good stuff.

- I saw changes pretty quickly, especially in the muscle I was gaining.

- I never felt bad, only good. I never felt like I was starving or miserable like you do on many diets where they cut everything out cold turkey.

And here are some other changes she noticed:

- My sleep improved drastically. I've had sleeping problems since I was a child and for the first time in probably forever, I stated getting six to seven hours of a sleep a night.

- I started feeling like myself again. Happy, motivated, less stressed. I definitely became more pleasant to be around.

- My anxiety decreased significantly (this was a big one for me).

- My productivity at work improved. Because of the changes I listed above, I was able to manage stress better, had more energy, and overall was able to be more productive and get more done.

Part IV

FIX YOUR SUGAR BRAIN

Chapter 12

STARVED FOR SEROTONIN

Sugar-Free Ways to Satiate the Craving for Sugar

Did you find out in Chapter 5 that you were hungry for serotonin? If so, you're very likely in the grip of chronic anxiety. Sometimes it's just a little worry about having to pack for a weekend trip ("What if I forget my travel clock! What if I oversleep?!"). Sometimes it's more significant dread about major deadlines or unpaid bills ("We could lose the house! The kids will have to leave their schools! I'm too old to get another job!"). Either way, if you're short on serotonin, life is one long series of unnerving challenges, and you're never completely sure that you'll be able to meet them—at least not to your own satisfaction.

Perhaps your serotonin shortage leads you into the seven pitfall thought patterns, in which anxious, obsessive, or pessimistic thoughts seem to take over your mind and your feelings. (We'll learn more about them in Chapter 14.) With a serotonin shortage, you reach for sugar. The pleasure pathways override the hypothal-amus's signals for physical hunger. As you become addicted to food, you shrink your brain—making change feel harder and more elusive. Suddenly you're locked into a downward spiral of anxiety, which depletes your serotonin, making you reach for sugar, which makes you more anxious, which further depletes your serotonin, which shrinks your brain . . .

Following are some typical worries that my serotonin-starved patients share with me. Do any of these anxiety-provoking thoughts sound familiar?

Other people have it easier than I do. Their lives are more together.

I'm so fat. Everyone is thinner than I am.

No one else has to think about every single bite—but I do, or I'll gain a ton. What is *wrong* with me?

My weight is so out of control. My job is probably in danger, too. And I'll never have a good relationship!

I wish I could reassure you that everyone has moments of feeling insecure, unattractive, and out of control—it is by no means just you. I wish I could reassure you, too, that your worries are not reliable guides to reality but only to the place where your mind and feelings go when you are starving for serotonin. Is it any wonder that you crave the comfort foods that help to boost your serotonin levels? You are simply trying to raise your sero-tonin levels by looking for sweets and simple carbs to ease your anxiety and give you at least a temporary infusion of calm. If you're short on serotonin, you're likely to gravitate toward foods made with sugar and flour: cakes, cookies, pasta, bread. Our goal is to help you find all the calm and comfort you deserve, but from healthier foods and activities.

Your Sugar Brain Fix Plan

When you start your program, you'll be nourishing your mind, body, and spirit with serotonin-boosting foods and activities. I want you to load yourself up with the following "S" words:

Sweet—Berries and other whole fruits can give you a boost of sweetness that can ease your cravings for sugar. They produce a slow and steady boost of serotonin in your brain and won't spike blood sugar the way sugar does.

Stretch—Choose calming exercises like yoga, Pilates, and simple daily stretching to cue your body to make more serotonin. Deep breathing, relaxing baths, and taking some quiet time are also great options. You can even use your serotonin-boosting foods to create a soothing experience—sip some chamomile tea while reading in bed.

Sleep—Did you know your body releases more ghrelin—the "hunger" hormone—when you don't get your seven or eight hours every night? Lack of sleep also interferes with your body's production of serotonin. A big mistake many of my patients make is falling asleep with the computer or television on. Their lights can disrupt your circadian rhythms, so unplug the electronics and sleep your way to weight loss!

Sun—The relaxing rays of warm sunshine can have a powerful serotonin-boosting effect. Twenty minutes of sunlight gives you a healthy boost of vitamin D, a booster that helps combat depression. Don't overdo it, though. Twenty minutes a day of being outside is enough to feel the benefit.

Soothing—The fragrance of lavender incense, the warmth of a crackling fire, and the peaceful calm of a walk can all boost your serotonin levels, as can a relaxing massage, a long bath, or a comforting talk with a friend.

Spiritual—Reconnecting to your life's purpose and feeling your place in the universe can breed a sense of peace and security like nothing else. Let your longing for serotonin remind you that your spiritual side is hungry, too. Find your own relationship to prayer, secular meditation, time in nature, or volunteer activities that allow you to experience your deepest connection with our planet and our world.

What about Portion Sizes?

Feel free to enjoy generous but reasonable portion sizes of healthy foods. The good news is that without excessive pitfall foods hijacking your brain chemistry, you will begin to sense when you need to eat and how much is based on actual physical hunger. Without the huge serotonin surge and blood sugar spike of sugar, it's far easier to eat reasonable portions. There's a reason people binge on bread and not broccoli. In general, booster foods help you to recalibrate your taste buds to prefer generous servings of whole fruits, vegetables, and omega-3-rich proteins. Most people will find that as they add new, exciting booster foods, they will experience a significant decrease in their desire for packaged pitfall snacks, which are usually mostly sugar and bad fats that shrink your brain.

Serotonin-Boosting Foods

The first step in your Sugar Brain Fix is adding serotonin-boosting foods to your diet. Remember that your brain needs the amino acid tryptophan along with folate, vitamin B_6, vitamin C, zinc, and magnesium to manufacture serotonin.

Tryptophan: chia seeds, sunflower seeds, flaxseeds, pistachios, cashews, almonds, hazelnuts, peanuts, soybeans, tofu, tempeh, cheese, beans, salmon, cod, perch, meat, eggs, yogurt, avocados, bananas, tamarind

Folate: spinach, brussels sprouts, kale, romaine lettuce, mushrooms, asparagus, bananas, melon, lemons, Swiss chard, broccoli, lentils, black beans, kidney beans, black-eyed peas

Vitamin B$_6$: carrots, spinach, peas, bananas, sunflower seeds, pistachios, lentils, chickpeas, salmon, shrimp, turkey, beef, pork

Vitamin C: red and yellow bell peppers, chili peppers, acerola, papaya, guava, kale, strawberries, raspberries, oranges, melon, grapefruit, tangerines, black currants, apricots, plums, parsley, kiwi, broccoli, spinach, cauliflower, brussels sprouts, lychee, elderberries, pineapple, garlic, limes, tomatoes

Zinc: oysters, flounder, sole, crab, beef, bison, lamb, pork, turkey, chicken, yogurt, pumpkin or squash seeds, baked beans, tempeh, lentils, kidney beans, chickpeas, black-eyed peas, split peas, pine nuts, peanuts, cashews, almonds, sunflower seeds, cashew butter, natural peanut butter, tofu

Magnesium: broccoli, squash, spinach, beet greens, collard greens, Swiss chard, cashews, almonds, sesame seeds, black beans, coffee, salmon, halibut

Serotonin-Boosting Activities

Through the 28 days of your Sugar Brain Fix, you'll also be adding booster activities to your daily life. Since low serotonin means high anxiety, be kind and gentle with yourself when deciding which activities on this list to try. Start out with those that sound pleasurable and easy. Once you've got your serotonin stabilized, some of the more challenging options here may no longer feel like they're out of reach. Just remember: Slow and steady wins the race!

- Adopt a rescue animal.
- Apologize.
- Arrange an outing to a movie or concert.
- Ask your barista how his or her day is.
- Ask your stressed co-worker if there's something you can do to help.
- Attend a 12-step meeting.
- Attend a class.
- Attend a religious service or Bible study.
- Balance your checkbook.
- Be honest.
- Become a Big Brother or Big Sister.
- Bird-watch.
- Bowl.
- Breathe deeply for five minutes.
- Bring a reusable bag to the store.
- Bring home one flower for your significant other . . . or yourself.
- Build a sand castle.
- Build a snowman.
- Call just to say "I love you."
- Canoe.
- Coach a kid's team.
- Cook.
- Cuddle with your significant other or pet.
- Do a crossword puzzle.
- Do a fasted workout.
- Do a favor and expect nothing in return.
- Do the dishes.
- Do your errands on foot or on your bike.
- Do your taxes.
- Eat dinner in the dark and taste every bite.
- Exercise.
- Fly a kite.
- Forgive.
- Garden.
- Get health insurance.
- Get or give a massage.
- Get rid of clutter.
- Get that mammogram or medical test you've been putting off.
- Give somebody a compliment.
- Give your pet a bath.
- Give yourself a compliment.
- Give yourself a face mask or scrub.

- Go a whole day without using your car.
- Go dancing.
- Go fishing.
- Go online and look at photos of foreign cities or landscapes.
- Go to a farmers' market.
- Go to a library or bookstore just to browse.
- Go to a museum.
- Go to a petting zoo.
- Go to a stand-up comedy show.
- Go to bed 30 minutes earlier than usual.
- Go to the opera or theater.
- Go to the top floor of a parking structure and take in the view.
- Golf.
- Half-smile for five minutes.
- Have a dance party with your kids.
- Have a good conversation.
- Have a TV- or computer-free evening.
- Hike a trail.
- Hold a baby.
- Hold a puppy.
- Hold hands.
- Hold the door for someone.
- Horseback ride.
- Hug somebody.
- Invite friends or family over just to chat.
- Jog.
- Join a support group.
- Journal—jot down what you're grateful for, any overwhelming feelings you'd like to unload, or any great ideas!
- Kayak.
- Knit.
- Let the person with just a few things go ahead of you at the store.
- Light a candle or incense.
- Listen to a friend's problems.
- Listen to classical or peaceful music.
- Look at old pictures.
- Look in the mirror and find one thing you like about the way you look.
- Look into someone's eyes when you're talking to them.

- Make a $5 donation to a charity online.
- Make amends.
- Make love.
- Meditate (download my serotonin-boosting meditation at drmikedow.com).
- Mow your lawn.
- Open a Facebook account and get in touch with an old friend.
- Open a savings account and plan for a trip you want to take.
- Organize your desk, closet, or junk drawer.
- Paint.
- Pamper yourself.
- Pay a bill.
- Pay for the person behind you at the tollbooth.
- Plan a potluck.
- Plan a surprise party.
- Plan for retirement.
- Play a game—with a team or by yourself.
- Play an instrument.
- Play with your pet.
- Practice tai chi/qigong.
- Pray.
- Put on warm socks.
- Quilt.
- Rake the leaves.
- Read.
- Recycle.
- Rub lotion on your hands or feet.
- Sail.
- Say hello to a stranger in the elevator.
- Say no when you need to, and don't feel guilty about it.
- Scrapbook.
- Send a card.
- Send somebody flowers.
- Set the table and sit down to eat.
- Sing along to the radio.
- Skip rocks.
- Skype with a faraway friend.
- Smell the roses . . . literally.
- Smile.
- Speak your truth.
- Spend a little time at a park or beach.
- Start a piggy bank.
- Stop and admire the view.

- Stretch for five minutes or more.
- Study.
- Sunbathe (wearing safe, planet-friendly, mineral-based sunblock).
- Swim.
- Take a bath.
- Take a small step toward achieving a big goal.
- Take a 20-minute nap.
- Take a walk—a brisk after-work stress reliever or a leisurely after-dinner stroll. Get the family involved!
- Take a yoga or Pilates class.
- Take deep breaths for several minutes while visualizing positive thoughts.
- Take photos—even if it's just with your cell phone.
- Take some old clothes to Goodwill or the Salvation Army.
- Take the stairs.
- Talk to a therapist.
- Tell a friend how much he or she means to you.
- Tell yourself three things you like about yourself.

- Treat yourself to a subscription to your favorite magazine.
- Try bright light therapy in the morning.
- Try positive visualization.
- Try my Subconscious Visualization Technique. (You'll find the practice in my book *Your Subconscious Brain Can Change Your Life* or videos at HayHouse.com.)
- Turn off your phone for one hour.
- Visit a loved one's grave and tell them why they'd be proud of you today.
- Volunteer.
- Walk or run for a cause.
- Walk your dog.
- Watch a funny or inspiring show on TV.
- Watch your favorite romantic comedy.
- Write a letter longhand, on paper.
- Write a poem.
- Write down your childhood dreams.
- Write your memoir.

Pitfall Foods

While you're stabilizing your serotonin by boosting activities and adding healthier foods in the weeks to come, you'll also need to be mindful of cutting back on the following pitfalls. Not to worry, because your serotonin will become balanced through other, sustainable sources of this feel-good chemical, which means you won't need to use sugar in one of its many forms. When that happens, eating fewer of these pitfall foods will start to feel effortless. When in doubt, check the label. As a reminder, "sugar" means all the foods that tend to be quickly converted into sugar or negatively affect blood sugar. Sugar in all its forms, artificial sweeteners, fruit juice (except lemon or lime), grains, and flour are all pitfall foods.

- Ace-K or acesulfame-K
- Agave nectar/syrup
- Amaranth
- Aspartame
- Barley
- Barley malt
- Beet sugar
- Blackstrap molasses
- Brown rice syrup
- Brown sugar
- Buckwheat
- Bulgur
- Buttered sugar/ buttercream
- Cane juice crystals
- Cane sugar
- Caramel
- Carob syrup
- Castor sugar
- Coconut sugar
- Confectioner's sugar (aka, powdered sugar)
- Corn syrup
- Corn syrup solids
- Crystalline fructose
- Date sugar
- Demerara sugar
- Dextrin
- Dextrose
- Diastatic malt
- Einkorn
- Equal
- Ethyl maltol
- Evaporated cane juice
- Farro
- Florida crystals

- Flour (all except almond, coconut, teff, and tigernut)
- Fructose
- Fruit juice (except lemon or lime)
- Fruit juice concentrate
- Galactose
- Golden sugar
- Golden syrup
- Glucose
- Glucose syrup solids
- Grape sugar
- Grains
- High-fructose corn syrup (HFCS)
- Honey
- Icing sugar
- Invert sugar
- Kamut
- Kaniwa
- Lactose
- Malt syrup
- Maltodextrin
- Maltose
- Maple syrup
- Millet
- Molasses
- Muscovado sugar
- Oats
- Panela sugar
- Quinoa
- Raw sugar
- Rice (all)
- Rice syrup
- Refiners syrup
- Saccharin
- Sorghum syrup
- Spelt
- Splenda
- Sucralose
- Sucrose
- Sugar (granulated or table)
- Sucanat
- Sunett
- Sweet One
- Sweet'N Low
- Turbinado sugar
- Treacle
- Wheat
- Yellow sugar

One Step at a Time

So now you know *what* you need to do. If you're like most serotonin-deprived people, *how* you do it will be just as important in your transformation process. Be forgiving with yourself, and always be on the lookout for what you did *right* today as opposed to focusing on what you did *wrong*. Some low-serotonin perfectionists will want to bypass gradual detox and shock their brains right into an all-brain-boosting-food regime beginning on day 1. Remember, this is probably the same perfectionism that has gotten you into trouble before!

When it comes to the lifelong journey of keeping your brain big and your waistline trim, it's a marathon, not a sprint. And the race is only with yourself. Since food can be addictive, the same catchphrases that apply to other addictions apply: "One day at time." "Easy does it." "Fake it till you make it." Remember: Low serotonin can trigger feelings of perfectionism, anxiety, self-criticism, and doubt to steer you off course. When you notice these feelings, sugar's seductive and destructive call tends to be particularly alluring. Instead of self-medicating with a brain-shrinking food, eat a serotonin-boosting food or choose an activity from this chapter. By doing so, you're helping your body to manufacture steady stores of soothing serotonin, which will leave you feeling fabulous and free.

Chapter 13

DOPAMINE DEPRIVED

"Kediterranean" Diet–Approved Ways to Satiate the Craving for Fat

If you discovered in Chapter 6 that you're low on dopamine, you may be frustrated with a life that seems too slow and boring, or you might have the opposite problem: feeling overwhelmed by a life that feels too fast and full. Maybe you bounce from deadline to deadline or crisis to crisis, always pulling out a little more energy, a few more reserves—only to feel burned out. Or perhaps you feel trapped in a dead-end job or in a narrow life, wondering how you ended up spending every waking minute on child care and housekeeping, with so little room for fun.

If the serotonin addict is an anxious eater, the dopamine addict is a depressed one. Feeling empty, lonely, or perhaps a little bit lost can all lead to self-medicating with bad fats that make dopamine surge. Plus, low-dopamine types are much more likely to avoid talking about feelings than those with low serotonin, so your friends may not know that you're unhappy or how frustrated and unfulfilled you are. You continue to overwhelm your brain with too many bad fats, bypassing signals for physical hunger. Over time, this shrinks the brain and makes change feel impossible.

Even if your life looks successful and put together, your dopamine deprivation may reflect some subtle problems that you're having trouble acknowledging, even to yourself. Maybe you and your partner are too tired for the kind of sex you'd like to have. Maybe you've mastered your formerly satisfying job and no longer find it a challenge. Maybe your wonderful kids fill your heart with love, but still you long for a bit of adventure.

Either way, if you're dopamine deprived, you are likely to crave genuine excitement to combat a growing sense of depression. Do any of the following thoughts and feelings sound familiar?

Is this all there is?

Surely life should hold more than this!

Where did all the fun and excitement go?

I haven't done anything new in a long time . . .

I don't recognize myself—how did I become so boring?!

I used to be a passionate person—what happened?

I want to help you awaken that part of yourself that feels stifled and suppressed by either boredom or too much work. Hopefully your Sugar Brain Fix will convince you to make the time and energy for yourself, and to commit to the pleasure in your life as much as you have already committed to your daily tasks and duties. You'll see that foods with bad fat, which trigger a short-term rush of dopamine, aren't adding any satisfaction to a life that might seem too stale. Our goal is to help you find all the thrills and adventure you crave—but from healthier foods and activities that help grow the brain.

Your Sugar Brain Fix Plan

When you start your program, you'll be nourishing your mind, body, and spirit with dopamine-boosting foods and activities. I want you to remind yourself of the following "D" words:

Deep-fried and fatty to lean and mean—If you're like most dopamine-deprived people, you will have gravitated to french fries, fried chicken, and energy drinks to give you the spark that you long for in your life. But there's another great source of dopamine, and that's protein filled with good fats such as omega-3-rich seafood and olive oil that's rich in monounsaturated fat. If you're dopamine deprived, you need protein—and lots of it. You should be sure to have some protein with every meal. Load up on omega-3-rich superfoods like seafood, beans, and oils.

Daring—You're craving change, excitement, and adventure, so mix it up by learning a new skill or doing something you've always dreamed about doing. Ski down a mountain, learn to parasail, ride in a hot-air balloon, or do some public speaking. Sign up for that online dating service, or ask that cute barista out for breakfast. Scare the hell out of yourself! The more adventure in your life, the less fat you'll crave. Even mix up your dopamine superbooster foods in daring ways. Scrambled organic eggs with broccoli and hot sauce may sound daunting to some, but not for you!

Delight—If we don't get delight in our lives, we'll look for it in our food. Marvel at a sunset, visit an intriguing new stretch of a neighborhood, spend 10 minutes a day doing something you love. You'll fill up on pleasure, and those french fries will just look like, well, greasy, brain-shrinking potatoes.

Desire—I can't advise you to fall in love—but if you did, it would be great for your brain! What about rekindling some romance with your significant other? Or, if you're single, do something you've always considered romantic, sexy, or thrilling: Visit Italy, learn to play poker, take a tango class. Find *something* you desire, and give yourself permission to pursue it.

Dare—Dopamine-deprived people need challenges, so test your creativity and see what you come up with. You might decide to redesign your garden, move around furniture in your living room or bedroom, or reorganize your closets. Learn a language, play competitive Scrabble, or pick up a book of sudoku—anything to experience a sense of struggle and accomplishment.

Dopamine-Boosting Foods

The first step in your plan is adding some of these dopamine-boosting foods to your diet. Remember that your body needs the amino acid tyrosine in combination with iron, vitamin C, and folate to manufacture dopamine. You don't have to eat all of these foods, but if you could find 10 or 20 you like, that'd be a great place to start. And since you're likely craving new adventures in your life, it won't be hard for you to try new foods. Maybe you could even challenge yourself by trying every food on this list. I dare you!

IF YOU FAIL TO PLAN, YOU PLAN TO FAIL

Since a shrunken brain and low dopamine are both associated with impulsivity, it's especially important for you to plan ahead. Have brain-boosting foods on hand when you come home in case you're in the habit of eating as soon as you walk in the door.

Tyrosine: fish, beef, lamb, pork, chicken, avocados, bananas, eggs, turkey, peanuts, almonds, pumpkin seeds, sesame seeds, lima beans, cheese

Iron: sardines, oysters, clams, mussels, liver, fish, pumpkin seeds, sesame seeds, squash seeds, nuts, broccoli, spinach, chicken, tofu, beef, turkey, ham

Vitamin C: red and yellow bell peppers, chili peppers, acerola, papaya, guava, kale, strawberries, raspberries, oranges, melon, grapefruit, tangerines, black currants, apricots, plums, parsley, kiwi, broccoli, spinach, cauliflower, brussels sprouts, lychee, elderberries, pineapple, garlic, limes, tomatoes

Folate: spinach, brussels sprouts, kale, romaine lettuce, mushrooms, asparagus, bananas, melon, lemons, Swiss chard, broccoli, lentils, black beans, kidney beans, black-eyed peas

Dopamine-Boosting Activities

Through the 28 days of the Sugar Brain Fix, you'll also be adding these booster activities to your daily life. Remember, you're the expert on yourself, and your feelings are information that indicate what you're needing at the moment. In the past, boredom would have mindlessly led you to a plate of chili cheese fries, but now you will be armed with a whole list of dopamine-boosting foods and activities you can use to fend off monotony.

Of course, have compassion toward yourself, and remember that low dopamine can be associated with hopelessness and sadness. So if this list of dopamine activities makes you feel overwhelmed, take a deep breath. Start slowly by adding five minutes of sudoku to your mundane Monday. Or treat yourself to a game night to shake up your weekend routine. As your dopamine levels begin to climb, so will your motivation to tackle more and more on this list—and in your life.

By using these activities instead of bad fats to get a natural hit of dopamine, they'll also help you with your transition to the Kediterranean diet.

- Act in community theater.
- Apply for a job.
- Ask a special someone on a date.
- Attend a 12-step meeting.
- Attend a lecture.
- Be the one to initiate sex tonight.
- Break down your list of goals into small, achievable subgoals.
- Browse realtor.com for a new house.
- Build something.
- Call in for a contest on a radio station.
- Clean the house at a quick pace to loud music.
- Cook something you've never made before.
- Dance.
- Do a fasted workout.
- Do some intense cardio or interval training.
- Do volunteer work that's rewarding and exciting.
- Drive a new way home from work.
- Dye your hair a new color . . . or let it go gray.
- Eat something you've never tried before.
- Fix something.
- Get a new haircut.
- Get eight hours of sleep.
- Get neurofeedback or EEG biofeedback.
- Get off at a train or bus stop in a part of town you've never been to before, or get in your car and drive to one.
- Get tickets to your favorite talk show or game show.
- Get waxed.
- Go ballroom dancing.
- Go Kart.
- Go shark tank diving.
- Go to a boot camp–style fitness class.
- Go to a city you've never been to before.
- Go to a restaurant you've never been to before.

- Go to a sporting event.
- Go to a zoo.
- Go to an open house just to look.
- Go to the target range.
- Go whitewater rafting.
- Go window shopping.
- Go wine tasting.
- Have a dance party with your kids.
- Have that conversation you've been meaning to have.
- Hike up a new trail.
- Hire a personal trainer.
- Hit some balls at a batting cage.
- Hit the playground with the kids.
- Host a theme party.
- Initiate foreplay.
- Invent something.
- Join a free meetup.com group—everything from hiking to groups just to meet new people.
- Join the PTA.
- Join Toastmasters, a public-speaking group.
- Jump off the diving board into the pool.
- Jump rope.

- Karaoke.
- Kiss.
- Learn a new language.
- Learn how to salsa.
- Lift weights.
- Make a movie on your phone.
- Make an obstacle course for the kids—see who can do it the fastest.
- Make love.
- Make some really hot salsa.
- Meditate (download my dopamine-boosting meditation at drmikedow.com).
- Miniature golf.
- Mountain bike.
- Order healthy takeout from a place you've never tried.
- Paint a room in your house a new color.
- Paint your nails a new color.
- Participate in a contest.
- Play a game or do a puzzle that challenges you, such as sudoku, a crossword puzzle, a video game, or poker.
- Play backgammon.

- Play ball.
- Play billiards.
- Play board games.
- Play bocce ball.
- Play darts.
- Play fetch with your dog.
- Play low-stakes poker with friends.
- Play Ping-Pong.
- Play soccer.
- Play tag.
- Play Twister.
- Poke around with one of those programs on your computer you've never used before.
- Read an exhilarating novel or story.
- Read the comics.
- Read your horoscope.
- Rearrange your furniture.
- Ride a roller coaster.
- Rollerblade.
- Sail.
- Scuba dive.
- See a therapist.
- Show up on time.
- Sign up for a dating website.
- Sign up for speed dating.

- Ski.
- Snorkel.
- Snowmobile.
- Spend five minutes browsing vacation spots online.
- Sprint.
- Start a blog.
- Start a fantasy football league.
- Submit your short story to a magazine.
- Surprise your significant other with a romantic fantasy.
- Surprise your significant other with some sexy lingerie.
- Take a belly dancing or pole dancing class.
- Take a cold shower.
- Take a spin class.
- Take a trapeze lesson.
- Take a walk in the rain.
- Take part in a flash mob.
- Take the stairs.
- Take your dog to the dog park.
- Test drive a new car— buy it only if you can afford it.

- Text somebody and tell them why you appreciate them.
- Train for a 5K.
- Try a new sport, such as fencing, tennis, or surfing.
- Try my Subconscious Visualization Technique. (You'll find the practice in my book *Your Subconscious Brain Can Change Your Life* or videos at HayHouse.com.)
- Try on a new pair of shoes.
- Vote.
- Walk a new path.
- Watch a game show.
- Watch a horror or action movie.
- Watch a street performer.
- Watch airplanes take off.
- Watch competitive sports—better yet, play one.
- Wear a new color of makeup today.
- Wear sexy underwear—even if it's just for you.
- Whiten your teeth.
- Write a song—and perform it for somebody.
- Write down five things you'd like to do this year.
- Write down 10 things you'd like to do in your life.

Pitfall Foods

As you boost your dopamine with booster foods and activities, you'll be cutting back on the pitfalls listed on the following page. You want to cut back on bad fats, which include industrial oils high in pro-inflammatory omega-6s, as you increase healthier oils. Stay away from the types of saturated fat that can shrink the brain like conventionally raised burgers or steak. Partially hydrogenated and trans fats are bad fats. As you know, a small amount of virgin coconut oil is permitted, especially if you're using it to help avoid a day of eating burgers.

Remember, as your dopamine levels begin to rise, these former pitfalls will start to lose their seductive lure. But that doesn't mean they're not problematic and potentially addictive, so it's important to keep them at arm's length. Do a pitfall food raid in your kitchen as you begin to stock up on foods that help you grow your brain. Especially with the impulsivity associated with a shrunken brain and low dopamine, it's important to make sure these foods aren't easily accessible in moments of weakness or boredom. I want you to really think about what you want to eat before it goes in your mouth. That way, these pitfall foods will become occasional treats, not perennial parts of your everyday life.

- Anything fried
- Anything in bad oils—which includes all oils except olive (all), virgin coconut, cold- or expeller-pressed canola, walnut, avocado, macadamia nut oil, Malaysian palm fruit oil
- All processed meats, including lunch meat—even white meat
- Conventionally raised/factory-farmed animal products, including meat, milk, eggs, and dairy

By Leaps and Bounds

Whenever we focus on our strengths, we are setting ourselves up for success and happiness. Dopamine-craving types need novelty, adventure, and challenges. Now that you are armed with an arsenal of ways to get these needs met in a healthy and sustainable manner, use that competitive streak in you to gradually yet powerfully commit to the life you know you want to live. It's not really about all the things you *can't* have; it's about getting what you really need so that the self-medicating substitutes fall by the wayside.

Chapter 14

THE POWER
OF THOUGHTS
AND BELIEFS

*Harnessing Your Subconscious
and Using Cognitive Behavioral
Therapy to Heal Your Sugar Brain*

One of my specialties is identifying thought patterns that lead to less-than-ideal moods and behaviors. Cognitive behavioral therapy (CBT) is rooted in this simple philosophy: Thinking in certain types of patterns makes us feel better, while thinking in other types of patterns makes us feel worse. I help my patients identify the thought patterns that get them into trouble and encourage them to reframe their thoughts into a more helpful approach. This helps them to rewrite their mantra—something you learned how to do in Chapters 5 and 6.

CBT is an integral part of the Sugar Brain Fix, because pitfall thoughts hurt your brain chemistry, lead to low levels of serotonin and dopamine, increase cravings for pitfall foods, shrink your brain, and then lead to more pitfall thoughts—another example of a downward spiral.

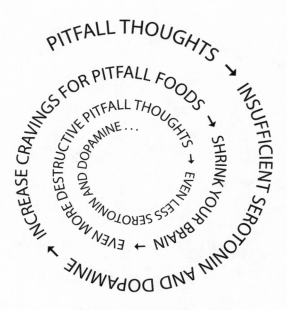

How do pitfall thoughts erode your stores of serotonin and dopamine? By feeding your anxiety, self-doubt, hopelessness, and despair, which leads to behaviors that cause more of these unpleasant feelings. Pitfall thoughts can make you feel helpless, worthless, and unsafe, and they can contribute to feeling stuck, trapped, and bored. If you have sugar brain, you're already feeling blue, stuck, impulsive, and/or foggy—so these pitfall thoughts take you from bad to worse. As we have seen, these are the feelings that accompany insufficient stores of serotonin and dopamine, which is precisely the brain-chemistry condition that sends you running for cheeseburgers and cheesecake to boost your mood. In fact, even if your diet is filled with terrific brain-boosting foods, pitfall thoughts can undo your good habits and push you toward your sugar or bad-fat fix.

Luckily, there is a way to reframe pitfall thoughts, so let me show you how it's done. We'll start by taking a close look at the seven pitfall thought patterns. Then, in the next section, I'll help you identify booster attributes that can raise your serotonin and dopamine levels—and fill your life with joy. Finally, at the end of this chapter, I'll show you how you can use self-hypnosis to heal your thoughts in an even more profound way.

The Seven Pitfall Thought Patterns

Pitfall #1: Personalization

Personalization is when you assume that something is happening because of you. Of course, sometimes you *are* responsible for a problem or a situation, and then you should realize that and own it. But the personalization pitfall comes into play when you have no explanation or another explanation, yet you still choose the one that involves blaming yourself.

Pitfall thoughts:

They didn't call me for an interview. I'm not smart enough.
He didn't call me because I'm too fat.
This diet isn't working because I have no self-control.

Reframed thoughts:

I really would have liked that job, so I'll keep looking. Perhaps they had already hired someone else.
I don't know why he didn't call me—maybe he's busy, insecure, or interested in someone else he met before me.
This diet isn't working—maybe it's time I did things differently and looked at what I need to change.

Here's how you can tell if you've personalized something: Just about every explanation for anything that goes wrong begins and ends with you not being good enough.

This kind of thinking can get you into trouble, because in pretty much any circumstance, you're usually only *one* part of the equation, and your shortcomings are only *one* part of you. Personalization blocks out all the aspects of life and relationships that are about other people or circumstances in general. Blaming yourself and taking things personally makes you feel hopeless, helpless, and unworthy.

Now, please don't start blaming yourself for taking things personally! Just try to reframe your thoughts to imagine other explanations. If you really want to avoid this pitfall thought pattern, try one week or even one day when you don't allow yourself to think of "not being good enough" as the reason for *anything.* You might be surprised at all the alternate explanations you come up with!

Pitfall #2: Pervasiveness

Pervasiveness is when any problem in any area of your life invades all the others. If one part of your life goes bad, you shut down in all areas. Naturally, this makes *everything* worse because you allowed one weakness to nullify all of your strengths.

Pitfall thoughts:

I gained some weight this week; I'm calling in sick to work tomorrow.
He didn't call me, so I'm not going to make an effort with him—or my friends, either.
I'm worried about money; I'm just going to pick up a pint of ice cream.

Reframed thoughts:

I gained some weight this week—but if I go into work tomorrow, I can have lunch with Maria, and she always cheers me up. I also know that once I'm there, I'll probably end up forgetting about most of my frustration.

He didn't call me, and it's times like these when my friendships are actually more important. Even though I don't really feel like it, I'm going to call a few friends and see if I can schedule some get-togethers.

I'm worried about money, but the last thing I want to do is be worried about money and *my health. I'm going to take a 10-minute walk and then focus on what financial changes I can make.*

When something goes wrong in one part of our lives, it's easy to let that affect *all* of our life. The antidote to pervasiveness is *perspective.* In the grand scheme of things, your sorrow, frustration, or failure, however painful or upsetting, is only one piece of your life. Don't let it spoil all the rest.

Some people believe that the antidote for pervasiveness is *gratitude.* They go by the maxim "I was upset that I had no shoes—until I met the man who had no feet." The point of remembering what you have to be grateful for is *not* to undermine your feelings or to mock you for having a hard time. It's to help you remember that there is always something more than the present moment, and always something greater than a single setback or even a whole period of setbacks. Reframing your pervasiveness into a larger vision of your life can help you boost your brain chemistry and regain your balance.

Pitfall #3: Paralysis by Analysis

This pitfall involves getting stuck in your own thoughts, trying to analyze what's wrong with you every time a sad, angry, or unpleasant feeling surfaces. Sometimes it's appropriate to try to figure out a problem or solve a difficult situation. But if you've thought about that problem all you can and either there isn't any solution or there isn't one that you can implement right away, sometimes it's simply better to distract yourself than to ruminate.

Pitfall thoughts:

What does it mean about me that I can't lose weight? I can't stop thinking about this.

I wonder if my co-worker is angry at me. I wonder why it took her so long to answer that e-mail today—what does that mean? Now that I'm thinking about it, there was also that other time last week when she gave me a strange look.

I'm feeling blue, and I'm going to sit here thinking about why until I feel better.

Reframed thoughts:

I've done all I can today to work on my weight-loss issues—now I'm going to take a bath and read a good book and forget about it! Tomorrow is a new day.

It's 8 P.M., and I'm spending my precious free time analyzing my work situation! I'm going to enjoy this beautiful night and take my dog for a walk before bed.

I'm feeling blue. I'm going to get up and do something productive instead of spinning around and around with all this negativity.

If you feel that you tend to get stuck in your own thoughts, here's my suggestion: Give yourself a time limit to think about something and set a timer. Check in with yourself when the timer rings and ask yourself honestly, "Am I making any progress in solving this problem?"

If the answer is no, say to yourself—aloud if necessary—"I can come back to this later." Then go do something else that will distract you from your thoughts. If you find this difficult, make a list of good "distractors," and when you get "paralysis by analysis," look at the list. The best antidote that helps people climb out of a deep hole of paralysis by analysis is doing something that will bring you a little pleasure or productivity. Who knows? Maybe the solution to your problem will come to you when you're busy doing something else—it often happens that way! Or maybe your problem *has* no solution, but you can feel better anyway.

Pitfall #4: Pessimism

Pessimism in this context means believing the worst-case, catastrophic scenario. If there is good evidence to think that something won't work or that danger is approaching, then by all means, take appropriate action. But when pessimism is your default response to any setback, it may be time to reframe your thoughts. Don't confuse what's possible with what's probable.

Pitfall thoughts:

I gained some weight this week. I can't make this work and I'm going to have a heart attack and die.

Relationships don't work out for me, so I bet this one won't, either. I'm going to be alone forever, and then what will I do when I'm 60?

I went on a job interview, but I'm sure I won't get this or any other job. What if I can't pay my mortgage next year?

Reframed thoughts:

I gained some weight this week, but I haven't really given this program a chance yet. Although it's possible that I could have a heart attack, I'm not experiencing any critical symptoms right now. I've also consulted my physician, and she said the best thing I can do for my health is lose weight.

I'm a different person than the last time I was in a relationship, so let's see what happens now.

I don't know whether I'll get the job or not, but I won't stop trying until I find something I like. Although it's possible I won't find a job for a whole year and lose the house, it's not probable. I've never gone more than three months without finding a job.

Pessimists are always imagining the worst-case scenario, in which any setback can easily be seen as the beginning of a catastrophe. This thinking leads to depression, anxiety, and despair. Optimists take a different approach: They imagine good possibilities that *might* happen, whether or not they ever do. Imagining these happy possibilities often gives optimists the energy to explore them, which means that optimists often end up creating good outcomes in their lives, simply because they were committed to finding a way to make the best of things or to see potential in a difficult situation. Whenever possible, they think, *Maybe it will be all right*, or *I'm sure there's some good that can come from this*—and frequently, because of their positive attitude, they see possibilities to pursue that pessimists might miss.

I'm not suggesting you become a Pollyanna, blind to genuine dangers or tragedies. But I do encourage you to develop an optimistic explanatory style and that you find a way of talking yourself out of pessimistic thinking, rather than deeper into it. Creating a "can-do, can-deal-with" attitude can really help you when times are tough.

Pitfall #5: Polarization

Polarization is seeing things in terms of either/or: black or white, yes or no, on or off. Instead of seeing that there are lots of possibilities, polarization is a pitfall in which you can imagine only *It's working* or *It's not working*. That means if something isn't working perfectly, you tend to believe it isn't working at all—and probably never will.

Pitfall thoughts:

I didn't lose weight this week—my whole diet is a failure. In fact, I should go on a different diet tomorrow.

If Terry doesn't understand this point, then this relationship is not going to work out.

Eating this one cookie has now ruined my entire day of healthy eating. I'm a total failure . . . I might as well go eat whatever I want for dinner. The day is totally ruined anyway.

Reframed thoughts:

I didn't lose weight this week—but I did two booster activities and feel like I made some healthy choices. I think I'm taking baby steps and making progress, even though I have a long way to go.

Terry and I clearly see things differently when it comes to this. But we do usually agree on things. Maybe this is going to have to be an "agree to disagree" situation. We love each other so much.

I did eat one cookie, but I filled the rest of my day with brain-boosting foods. Overall, I'd give this day a B+. Not bad! I'm going to continue the progress with a delicious brain-boosting dinner!

Giving up polarization does not mean that you stop taking negative factors into account. It means that you put them in context. When we're trying to make lots of changes, we often take two steps forward and one step backward, or sometimes even one step forward and *two* steps backward. Seeing the situation in a polarized way means we're far too excited about the progress—and then far too disappointed when we take that backward step. If we can reframe our thinking to accommodate all the different possibilities, we can operate on a more even keel.

Pitfall #6: Psychic

This is the frame of mind in which we're sure we know what another person is thinking, we believe *he* should know what *we're* thinking, and we also think we know the future. In other words, we are *sure* of a lot of things that we actually can't really know.

Pitfall thoughts:

If he cared about me, he'd see I was struggling and help me by eating healthy foods with me.

I don't think my friend likes me anymore. She hasn't texted in weeks.

I know if I go, everyone will be thinking how fat I am.

Reframed thoughts:

I'm going to tell him just how hard this really is for me, and I bet if I asked him to support me by trying a few booster foods, too, he would.

I'm going to reach out to my friend. She hasn't said that she doesn't like me and nothing has really changed. If we spend a little time together, we'll reconnect—and if I still sense something is wrong, I'll ask her.

I feel self-conscious, but I have no idea what other people are thinking about me or even if they're thinking about me at all.

Giving up our "psychic" pitfall thinking can be very difficult because it often feels as though we're giving up our claim to know the truth and to protect ourselves. Sometimes our instincts are right on target and we have to listen to them; sometimes another person has hurt or disappointed us repeatedly, and we have to protect ourselves from trusting them again.

Sometimes, though, we're just living inside our own fears, wishes, and projections, and what we "know" is not the truth at all but merely a story we've imagined. Being rigorous with yourself about what you know and don't know—or at least about being open to the possibility that you might not know—is a good antidote for this pitfall. Committing to telling other people very clearly what we're feeling or asking others what's on their minds is another good reframing device.

Pitfall #7: Permanence

Another name for this pitfall is "using the past to judge the future." I personally struggle a lot with this one. If I try something a few times and it doesn't work out, I have a hard time believing that it will *ever* work out, even when logic and rationality tell me that I'm giving up way too soon. I'm also prone to think, *I've always been this way—I can't change,* even though I have the privilege of watching people's transformations every single day in my practice.

Pitfall thoughts:

I've never been able to lose weight, so I'm just doomed to be fat forever.

I feel so sad and lonely. I'm always going to feel like this. This will never pass.

I've never had a management job—I guess I'm going to be stuck in this job forever.

Reframed thoughts:

Although I've never lost weight before, I've found a new approach to eating that just might work.

Even though I feel sad and lonely right now, I'm doing things to change it. I remember feeling this way 10 years ago, and even though things looked just as bad then, I did get out of that funk.

Just because I don't have that management job now doesn't mean that I'll never have it. I'm going to do everything I can to increase the likelihood that I'll get the next one that opens up.

It's very tempting to judge the future by the past, especially because that makes us the expert. We *know* what happened in the past, so now we can *know* what's going to happen in the future. We can protect ourselves from disappointment and maybe even avoid the hard work of transformation and growth.

I urge you to resist the lure of the "permanence" pitfall. Instead, accept that the future is unknown and that you have both the opportunity and the responsibility to create the life you want.

The Seven Booster Qualities

Just as pitfall thoughts erode your brain chemistry, booster qualities *improve* your brain chemistry. In fact, the more of these booster qualities you fill your life with, the fewer pitfall thoughts you will have. All the booster activities target one or more of these booster qualities, so by the end of 28 days, you will look back and realize your serotonin- or dopamine-boosting activities have created a life rich with these seven booster qualities. It's also easier to sustain booster qualities when you have sufficient serotonin and dopamine—a nice example of an *upward* spiral!

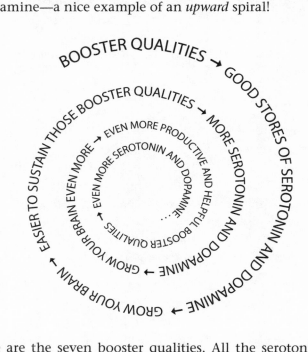

Here are the seven booster qualities. All the serotonin- and dopamine-boosting activities will add one of these qualities to your life. As you read this list, ask yourself: Which booster quality do I need more of in my life right now?

Booster Quality #1: Purpose

Filling our lives with purpose is the best way to cultivate lasting and meaningful happiness. Why are you here? What's your life's purpose on this planet? What do you think you'll remember most when you're looking back on your life? My guess is that you'll remember your relationships, the times you made a difference in the world—even on a small scale—and the work you did, paid or unpaid, that was your chance to express yourself. These things have the greatest impact on your well-being and lasting happiness. They are also the behaviors that give you lasting surges of serotonin and dopamine. If you can switch from asking "What do I want out of life?" to asking "What does life want out of me?" you may be surprised at how rich and full of possibilities your life suddenly seems.

Booster Quality #2: Peace

What fills your life with a sense of peace or calm? And what spiritual beliefs help you to make sense of your life? As you think about the answers to these questions, consider the practices that are both spiritual *and* good for your serotonin: meditation, yoga, prayer, listening to music. Filling our lives with peace also has a direct effect on weight. A lack of peace increases the stress hormone cortisol in the brain, which tells the body to store fat in the most dangerous place—the belly. So find the activity, the rescue animal, the relationship—along with the food—that help you bring peace into your life.

Booster Quality #3: Pride

If someone were to ask you, "What are the three things in your life that you are most proud of?" what would your answer be? When you can feel good about these answers, your serotonin and dopamine stores will rise. Enjoy the qualities and achievements that you are most proud of—revel in them and share them with others—and your brain chemistry and your waistline will benefit.

Booster Quality #4: Power

What gives you a sense of power in your life? People who don't feel power are prone to hopelessness, anger, low self-worth, and sadness. We all need to feel powerful, to experience a sense of competency and mastery in some part of our lives. You can increase your sense of power by knowing you are a good parent or that you are really good at sudoku. You can know you're a good driver, and when you use that skill to volunteer for a Meals on Wheels program, well, then you really have a double whammy in feeling good. Your serotonin and dopamine levels rise, and you feel empowered to make changes in your diet and your health. But if you don't think you're good at *anything,* then everything becomes harder. Ask yourself, "What are my strengths, and how can I best use them?" In that answer lies your power.

Booster Quality #5: Passion

What are the things in this world that truly interest you? You usually know it by your perception of time: When you're engaged in an activity you're passionate about, time seems to fly by. No two people are alike, so it's important to fill your life with things that are captivating to *you*. When we operate from this approach, our lives feel more fulfilling. We actually *want* to read up about a topic or spend our time with that hobby. You can find passion in many places—work, relationships, hobbies, or volunteer opportunities. What happens when we have this in our lives? You guessed it: hefty doses of dopamine in the brain, since engaging in activities you're passionate about is rewarding.

Booster Quality #6: Productivity

One of the best things we can do when we feel sad is to distract ourselves with something that makes us feel productive. Clean out that junk drawer. Go to work. Do the laundry. Even if you don't feel like it . . . *especially* when you don't feel like it. This sort of redirection helps to decrease many pitfalls in our life, particularly paralysis by analysis, pervasiveness, and pessimism. Being productive builds our brain chemistry as it helps us to take action in our lives and instill a sense of purpose. Our serotonin increases, because we have more positive things to focus on.

Booster Quality #7: Pleasure

Pleasure, dopamine, and serotonin go together like ice cream and hot fudge—or like berries and organic Greek yogurt. So when you're sad, get a massage! Watch your favorite TV show. Laugh. All of these are great serotonin and dopamine boosters, and maybe just the thing you need to feel good. But remember, a truly happy and healthy life has a balance of all these boosters—so don't get stuck living a life of just pleasure!

The Power of Hypnosis

Amber had tried everything. Support groups, calorie-restricted meal delivery, food logs, nutritionists, personal trainers, and even a prescription medication to change her diet. All of them had helped her somewhat, but none of them resulted in sustainable, long-term change.

Amber was intrigued by the way self-hypnosis could rewire the brain. That's why it's famous for helping people to quit smoking—another deeply ingrained, hard-to-change habit.

"I don't know much about hypnosis, but something tells me that it's that missing piece I've been looking for!" she said with a look of optimism on her face. "If self-hypnosis can help people quit smoking, I think it could work for me to finally stop eating these foods I feel powerless over."

As I explained how self-hypnosis works, I could see her getting visibly excited. The subconscious is extremely effective at targeting deeply rooted patterns of behavior. After all, so many triggers and cravings for unhealthy food operate underneath our conscious awareness. The more sugar and bad fats shrink the brain, the more elusive change can be. That's where the power of self-hypnosis comes into play. Changes made with the subconscious feel different than those made through conscious channels.

A unique skill of the subconscious is that it can access memories and the emotional centers of your brain far more quickly and effectively than the conscious. By accessing memories that may be linked to eating and erasing triggers to self-medicate with brain-shrinking food, change starts to feel possible. Visualizing changes via self-hypnosis can even trick the brain into believing the change has already occurred. If a change has already happened, it means that it's possible.

"When you've used other behavioral change strategies, you're using conscious strategies to create change. When you do that, you have to strong-arm changes in your behavior—in ways that feel calculated and rational," I explained to Amber. "By accessing the subconscious through self-hypnosis, change often begins to happen rapidly and effortlessly."

"*That* would be incredible," she said with excitement, "because even when I find something that works, it feels so hard."

"If we can *add* self-hypnosis to your toolbox, I have a feeling you're going to be successful in creating change that lasts. Let's supercharge your efforts with a little magic from your subconscious brain."

Amber looked at me and had a genuine smile on her face. "I can't wait!"

What Is Self-Hypnosis?

Self-hypnosis isn't going to make you bark like a dog. It won't brainwash you. Your willingness is required. Like a meditation practice, you'll go deeper the more you use it. The deeper you go, the more effective—and even magical—it will feel.

Self-hypnosis taps into the wonder of your subconscious. What exactly *is* the subconscious? The *Oxford English Dictionary* defines the subconscious as "the part of the mind of which one is not fully aware but which influences one's actions and feelings." Another helpful definition from the Collins dictionary says the subconscious is "that part of the mind which is on the fringe of consciousness and contains material of which it is possible to become aware by redirecting attention."

To fix sugar brain, self-hypnosis is a fantastic add-on to the cognitive behavioral tools you just learned how to use in the last chapter—like identifying the pitfall thought patterns that fuel unhealthy eating. Self-hypnosis creates a unique state of heightened absorption and concentration that's sometimes referred to as trance, and this trance state can help you take changes even further. For example, self-hypnosis helps some people find forgotten childhood memories that helped create pitfall thought patterns and addiction to brain-shrinking foods. Others find it deletes triggers for unhealthy foods as it installs positive self-talk. You're more likely to accept positive suggestions, including those to eat brain-healthy foods, when you're in a trance.

Trance is simply an altered state of mind. We can use food, drugs, or alcohol to create trance states. But you can also learn to use self-hypnosis to create a trance state simply by harnessing the power of your mind.

Studies have shown the combination of cognitive behavioral therapy (CBT) and self-hypnosis to be a true powerhouse. Researchers looked at all the weight-loss studies that used self-hypnosis in combination with CBT. They calculated how many pounds, on average, subjects lost with cognitive behavioral therapy alone. Then they calculated how many pounds subjects who used CBT *with* hypnosis lost. The results? People who used hypnosis with CBT lost *twice* as much weight compared to people using CBT by itself.

How exactly does self-hypnosis do this? Many of the spells it weaves are thanks to the magic of the scientifically proven theta brainwave. Your brainwaves can be measured as electricity on an EEG. From fastest to slowest, your brainwaves are gamma, beta, alpha, theta, and delta. The aha moment that hits you all of a sudden is a fast gamma brainwave. When you're working on a spreadsheet, that's beta. When you relax or meditate, your brain is in alpha. When you're dreaming at night or using self-hypnosis, your brain has slowed down to theta. When you're in deep, dreamless sleep, that's delta.

The other way to understand the magic of self-hypnosis is in how it activates, deactivates, and rewires different brain structures. When I say *your subconscious brain*, I'm talking about this footprint that can be measured by brain imaging studies like functional MRIs and SPECT scans.

I had my own brain examined to put hypnosis to the test. I asked my friend and world-famous SPECT scan expert Dr. Daniel Amen to do both an EEG and SPECT on my brain. We did a baseline EEG and SPECT scan while I did nothing. Then we did a second EEG and SPECT scan while hypnosis activated my subconscious brain.

In terms of brainwaves, there was an overall increase in theta brainwaves. This explains the deep, dreamlike state. While most of my brainwaves were slowing down, there was an increase in fast, beta brainwaves in my brain's occipital lobe. This means that hypnosis was tricking my brain into believing it was actually seeing the things I was visualizing in my mind's eye. To fix sugar brain, you can see all sorts of things that can help you to grow your brain—from eating foods that help to maintain healthy brain chemistry to doing fasted workouts.

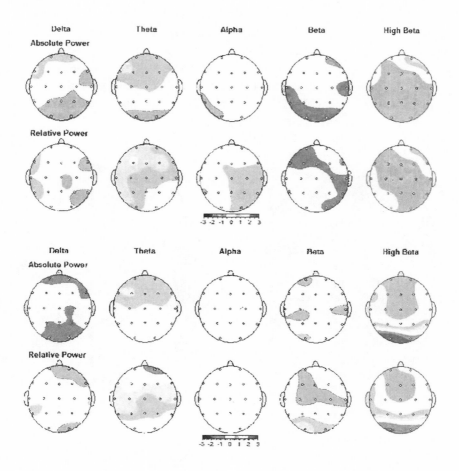

In terms of blood flow and activity, the SPECT scan showed hypnosis changed blood flow and activity in two parts of my brain. Hypnosis lit up my prefrontal cortex—the most advanced and "human" part of the brain. It's involved in planning, attention, and complex decision making. If you light up this part of the brain, it may feel easier to put the brakes on urges to eat brain-shrinking foods. The SPECT scan also showed hypnosis activated my basal ganglia. Because of all the dopamine released in this part of the brain, emotions, learning, and any behavior that affects reward systems—like eating—are affected. With self-hypnosis, you can

learn how to access feel-good states without needing to put anything in your mouth. By visualizing all the times in your life you
felt happy, you'll probably realize that you don't need sugar and
bad fats to release serotonin and dopamine. All the booster activities you'll add during the Sugar Brain Fix will add pleasure and
peace to your life while my Kediterranean diet–based program will
help you to eat brain-boosting foods.

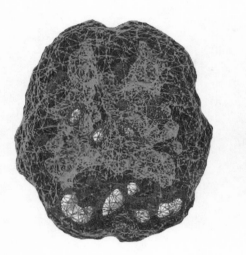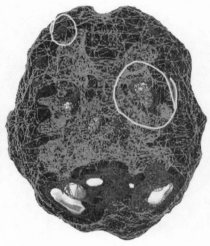

Self-hypnosis is also a powerful tool in helping you to connect
with and change bodily functions. This, of course, is incredibly
helpful when it comes to changing the way you eat. Scientists
suspect the power of self-hypnosis to change the body is due to
an increased connection between two parts of your brain when
you use this tool: the prefrontal cortex and insula. I've found that
many people with sugar brain are completely cut off from their
bodies when eating. Eating becomes mindless, and the serotonin
and dopamine from the brain-shrinking foods fuel this problematic behavior. The good news: You can use self-hypnosis to
reverse this.

You're Already Using Your Subconscious Brain

Even if you don't practice self-hypnosis, you're already using your subconscious brain all the time. When you're daydreaming, you're using your subconscious. If you're in a meeting, your conscious brain would be the one paying attention to what's being said. But let's say you get bored. Well, it's your subconscious that takes you somewhere fun in your mind's eye as a way to deal with boredom. Your subconscious also helps you to become immersed in plays, movies, and books.

If you've ever had the experience of barely remembering how you got home from your office or the store as you pulled into the garage, it was your *subconscious* taking over the wheel as your conscious was busy thinking about something. Or, perhaps a name escaped you. Despite trying your hardest to remember it, your conscious brain couldn't retrieve what you were seeking. Over the course of a day, your conscious brain was listening to your boss at a meeting, then typing up a Word document, and then making plans via text. But this whole time, your subconscious suddenly delivers that name that had escaped you hours earlier. Your subconscious brain is already helping you in your daily life, so self-hypnosis is simply a way for you to tap into a skill you already have been using.

WHO SHOULDN'T USE SELF-HYPNOSIS

The following script and audio track will help you to use self-hypnosis as a self-guided tool. This is not a substitute for the treatment of diseases that require professional help (e.g., anorexia, drug addiction). People with an untreated major dissociative disorder (e.g., dissociative amnesia, dissociative identity disorder, depersonalization-derealization disorder) shouldn't use self-hypnosis. These disorders require a professional and customized hypnosis scripts. Also, don't use self-hypnosis to recall or edit memories that may be the subject of legal proceedings. It's so powerful at helping you to edit your own memories that your testimony could possibly be deemed inadmissible in court.

Activating Your Subconscious to Help Fix Your Sugar Brain

If you'd like a little extra boost to help fix your sugar brain, add this self-hypnosis script. There's an audio download of this script included with this book. Use the script (or download) on day 1 of the 28-day program. If you'd like, you can also use it right now—before you start your journey. Then use it at least a few times per week throughout the program.

To go even deeper as you work to overcome the cravings for sugar and bad fats—and the feeling of being blue, stuck, impulsive, and foggy that come with sugar brain—you can take advantage of the video-enhanced self-hypnosis program that I put together. This program contains a variety of different self-hypnosis practices that have been combined with video that includes affirmations aimed at planting positive change. It also features set two-week programs to help you make self-hypnosis a natural and easy part of your routine. This program is available for purchase at www.HayHouseU.com.

Remember that self-hypnosis is a practice, just like meditation. The more you use self-hypnosis, the more you're shifting your body from a fight-or-flight state into a relaxed one. The peaceful feeling it creates prevents stress eating, and this is especially true for people who are short on serotonin. Self-hypnosis can also help you get a little dopamine boost as you visualize excitement with your mind's eye, making it a wonderful tool for people who are short on this activating neurotransmitter. For the Sugar Brain Fix program, practicing self-hypnosis can count as either a serotonin- or dopamine-boosting activity.

Starting out, I suggest you use this practice just before bed. If it makes you feel drowsy, you can drift off to sleep. You can also skip the re-alerting sequence at the end of the script if you'd like to go directly from the practice to bed. Your brain will naturally speed itself back up in the morning—just as it does every morning.

If you're using self-hypnosis in the middle of the day, be sure to use the re-alerting sequence at the end of the script. Make sure you're fully awake and alert before returning back to work or driving. Here's an abridged self-hypnosis script you can read. Listen to the full audio version of this practice with the link included at the end of this book. Using this practice can count as one of your booster activities once you begin the program.

I invite you to begin this practice by allowing the eyes to close as you settle in here . . . as the body finds the most comfortable position to rest. And as you settle here, make any last adjustments if you'd like, resting into this peaceful and pleasurable state. . . . I wonder if you can bring your attention to the place in the body where you feel the most relaxed. You already know how to activate the subconscious, which has always been here conspiring in your favor, so I invite you to begin this journey simply with some mindfulness. Ever so easily invite yourself to simply notice what's on your mind—right here and right now.

And now use the power of your mind's eye to imagine you're watching a parade . . . and this parade is made up of your thoughts . . . your feelings . . . your urges to engage in any habit that's not in alignment with your healthiest and highest self. . . . Isn't it nice to watch them float on by . . . without having to act on them? If you'd like, you could even picture a grand master leading the parade out from your brain through a path out of the ear to a place just in front of you . . . but here you are, watching from the sidelines . . . and feeling so peaceful.

Isn't it so nice to know that you don't have to join the parade . . . no matter where you see the grand master leading it? I wonder if that makes you feel a bit proud of yourself . . . or even more peaceful, perhaps. Many people find it so freeing to know that they don't have to act on these thoughts . . . these feelings . . . these urges . . . you can just watch as the parade passes by.

I wonder if you're even a little amused at how silly this parade can be at times . . . as all our parades tend to be. What do you see? Are people dressed in ridiculous costumes . . . or are there wild animals? I don't know exactly what you'll see in your parade . . . and it really doesn't matter . . .

What matters is whether you can bring a lightness to the way you greet your parade. Can you smile a bit now? Because the train that your subconscious brain is about to show you— and the places that your future self can take you—is far more impressive, isn't it? Oh, the places you will go. Would you like to take a peek? Who would want to board the fast train to nowhere when they could have a first-class ticket to Naples, Nice, or Norway?

Now pivot your attention to sounds, and invite the ears to notice three sounds you're hearing—right here and right now. That's right. It could be interesting to begin with the loudest sound you can perceive in this moment. And now find a noise that's neither loud nor soft—a medium sound. Now I wonder what's the quietest sound you can hear . . . can you hear your breath? That's right. Perfect.

And now invite the eyes to notice two colors you can see on the backs of the eyelids. The first being directly in front of you . . . and then, on the next inhale, what color can you see near the crown of the head as you roll the eyes up, up, up?

On the next exhale, allow the eyes to float down, down, down . . . and just relax the eyes now as you allow any lingering tightness to float away. Yes, that's right. And now I invite you to really feel one breath—allowing the breath to breathe you. Can you feel the breath rocking you? Can you feel the place where the breath feels the most pleasant or the most peaceful? Allow that feel-good or soothing sensation to spread through the brain and body. That's right. Perfect.

And now I invite you to take the next step by asking the subconscious to help you in the way you need it most today. Isn't it so nice to know that you already have the tools within you to change? By giving yourself this time today, you have already shown that you are honest, open, and willing, haven't you? I wonder what will show up for you today. . . . I don't know if it will complement all the tools you already use or if it will help you find some new ones . . . but what I do know is that it will help you find that deep part of you that knows that you are okay . . . that you are innately worthy . . . and as you begin to find pleasure in the simple things, you'll feel this peace and pleasure in ways that are in line with your highest self.

And now, focus on your inhales. Every inhale can take you back up to your everyday, awake, and alert state. That's right . . . as you give a little wiggle to your fingers and your toes, you can feel more and more rejuvenated. So refreshed and restored.

To ensure you're fully conscious again, look around the room and name aloud 10 items you see, take a walk around the block, listen to some upbeat music, or do 25 jumping jacks.

Now you understand how the Sugar Brain Fix will help you grow your brain and shrink your waistline. Self-hypnosis is now another tool you can add to your belt—one of many you'll be using during your 28-day journey. Now, it's time for the fun part: getting started!

Chapter 15

THE SUGAR BRAIN FIX PROGRAM

Now you're ready to start adding delicious booster foods and activities to your life! Here's the gradual detox portion of the Sugar Brain Fix program, which has you loading up on brain-boosting foods and then—when you are starting to get what you need from your life—gradually cutting out pitfalls. To find suggestions of booster activities, see pages 191 and 203.

Whether you're deficient in serotonin, dopamine, or both, all the pitfall foods in both these lists will count as a pitfall. A summary of pitfall foods: sugar, flour, fruit juice, grains, artificial sweeteners, industrial oils, processed meat, anything fried, and factory-farmed animal products.

As you already know, pitfall foods flood the brain with unsustainable amounts of serotonin and dopamine through sugar and bad fats, leading to a shrunken brain and an expanded waistline. Yes, they are as bad for your brain as they are for your body!

Brain-boosting foods give your brain sustainable energy by promoting a healthy release of serotonin and dopamine, which is, of course, good for both brain and body. They prevent inflammation in the brain and prevent it from shrinking. Intermittent fasting and fasted workouts increase the growth hormone BDNF to help you grow your brain and create new brain cells. Booster activities also promote healthy serotonin and dopamine levels, which will help you to decrease emotional eating and promote eating based on physical hunger. The hypothalamus in the brain can do its job and help you eat when you're hungry. A larger hippocampus can help you to feel better, control impulses, be hopeful, and remember every food you eat—increasing the time between meals and helping you to decrease the quantity of food you're eating. This combination of boosting will balance your brain chemistry and, yes, you will actually begin to favor and even crave foods that support brain health while feeling both physically and emotionally satisfied.

As you begin the program, the seven servings of vegetables and whole fruits will ensure that you're getting enough of the vitamins and minerals you need to create serotonin and dopamine from the amino acids in your diet. The daily omega-3 source will help you to tame inflammation and keep the brain in tip-top shape. Armed with the knowledge of which foods are particularly good for your brain chemistry, those who are low in serotonin can always favor foods with tryptophan. Also, you can favor them when you're feeling anxious or stressed out. Those who are low in dopamine can always favor foods rich in tyrosine. Reach for these foods when you're feeling low and need a pick-me-up. Those who are low in both neurotransmitters can alternate between tryptophan- and tyrosine-rich foods.

Serotonin- and dopamine-boosting foods have a lot more going for them than being healthy foods overall. They are also packed with one or more of the following healthy brain chemistry–promoting compounds: B vitamins, amino acids, omega-3s, and protective antioxidants. For example, salmon—especially wild-caught—is a protein with fat, which means it helps to release dopamine, but it also contains so many brain-nourishing omega-3s that it's good for increasing *both* serotonin and dopamine production. Blueberries, especially organic ones, have healthy levels of natural serotonin-boosting carbohydrates, but they also have antioxidants that prevent damage to your neurons—helping them to continue pumping both serotonin and dopamine. Check out Appendix A for some of my favorite brain-boosting recipes. These tools will help you make the booster food lists your grocery store list!

WEEK 1

Don't cut any foods out of your normal diet. Remember, we add before we take away.

Eat at least *seven* servings of whole fruits and vegetables. These will ensure you're getting the vitamins and minerals needed to manufacture serotonin and dopamine while keeping your brain big and beautiful.

Eat at least *one* omega-3-rich food every day. This will ensure you're getting more brain-boosting, anti-inflammatory fats.

Skip or replace *one* breakfast or dinner this week. You can either skip the meal altogether or replace it with bone broth or vegan broth.

Do *one* fasted-state workout. Work out just before the meal that comes after the one you skipped or replaced.

Add *one* boosting activity each day. Based on your findings in Part II, I gave you a list of activities that will replenish the neurochemicals you need most. If you need to replenish both serotonin and dopamine, alternate by adding a serotonin booster one day and a dopamine booster the next.

If you'd like, use the self-hypnosis audio track at least two times this week.

WEEK 2

Don't cut any foods out of your normal diet.

Eat at least *seven* servings of whole fruits and vegetables. These will ensure you're getting the vitamins and minerals needed to manufacture serotonin and dopamine while keeping your brain big and beautiful.

Eat at least *one* omega-3-rich food every day. This will ensure you're getting more brain-boosting, anti-inflammatory fats.

Skip or replace *two* meals this week. You can either skip these two meals altogether or replace them with broth. You can either skip or replace one dinner and the next morning's breakfast, or skip or replace two nonconsecutive meals: one breakfast and one dinner; two breakfasts; or two dinners.

Do at least *one* fasted-state workout. Work out just before the meal that comes after one you have skipped or replaced.

Add *two* serotonin- or dopamine-boosting activities each day. As with your food boosters, if you're both serotonin and dopamine deficient, add one booster activity for each neurochemical every day.

If you'd like, use the self-hypnosis audio track at least two times this week.

WEEK 3

Limit your pitfall foods to no more than *three* servings per day. A pitfall food serving should be around 300 calories at most, so you're going for a maximum of about 900 calories from foods made with brain-shrinking sugar (in all its forms) and bad fats.

Eat at least *seven* servings of whole fruits and vegetables. These will ensure you're getting the vitamins and minerals needed to manufacture serotonin and dopamine while keeping your brain big and beautiful.

Eat at least *one* omega-3-rich food every day. This will ensure you're getting more brain-boosting, anti-inflammatory fats.

Skip or replace *three* meals this week. Skip or replace one dinner and the next morning's breakfast plus one additional breakfast or dinner. If this is too difficult, you can skip or replace three nonconsecutive meals: three breakfasts; three dinners; two breakfasts and one dinner; or one breakfast and two dinners.

Do at least *two* fasted-state workouts. Work out just before the meal that comes after one you have skipped or replaced.

Add *three* serotonin- or dopamine-boosting activities each day. If you need to replenish both types of brain chemical, alternate between adding two serotonin boosters and one dopamine booster, and adding one serotonin booster and two dopamine boosters.

If you'd like, use the self-hypnosis audio track at least two times this week.

WEEK 4

Limit your pitfall foods to no more than *two* servings per day. Remember, one serving of a pitfall is about 300 calories, so you're looking at a maximum of about 600 calories of foods made from brain-shrinking sugar (in all its forms) and bad fats.

Eat at least *seven* servings of whole fruits and vegetables. These will ensure you're getting the vitamins and minerals needed to manufacture serotonin and dopamine while keeping your brain big and beautiful.

Eat at least *one* omega-3-rich food every day. This will ensure you're getting more brain-boosting, anti-inflammatory fats.

Skip or replace *four* meals this week. Skip or replace one dinner and the next morning's breakfast twice this week. Or, skip or replace one dinner and the next morning's breakfast plus two additional nonconsecutive breakfasts or dinners. Or, skip or replace four nonconsecutive meals: four breakfasts; four dinners; or a combination of breakfasts or dinners.

Do at least *two* fasted-state workouts. Work out just before the meal that comes after one you have skipped or replaced.

Add *four* serotonin- or dopamine-boosting activities each day. If you need to replenish both types of brain chemical, add two boosters of each type every day.

If you'd like, use the self-hypnosis audio track at least two times this week.

MAINTENANCE

Follow the program you followed in week 4.

Journal Your Way to Weight Loss

One of the simplest and clinically most effective ways to lose weight is to keep a food journal. You will be adding accountability to each meal and snack by writing down everything you consume, helping you to become more mindful and less likely to choose impulsively.

The Sugar Brain Fix journal has some other key elements. First, you will be tracking booster activities, fasting schedule, and workouts in addition to your food. You will also be writing about the way your daily efforts to balance your brain chemicals positively affect your mantra and your mood. This will help you feel motivated to keep on growing your brain as you give up all those brain-shrinking sugars and bad fats. This improvement in the way you feel is the ultimate reward, and this positive feedback will help you to keep your life going in the upward spiral you've created. The more you grow your brain, the easier these changes continue to feel. If you've felt that your mood is entirely out of your control, writing about your activities and their results will give you a sense of hope, as most of your mood is actually in your control, based on your daily choices to take care of your health, your body, and your life. Journaling will help you to bypass the fogginess, the impulsiveness, and the blues associated with sugar brain.

The Sugar Brain Fix: Frequently Asked Questions

Q. What if I really love pasta?

A. Swap out pasta for spiralized veggies. Or, find a pasta that's made only from beans or chickpeas.

Q. What about milk?

A. Favor unsweetened nut milks, which don't count as a pitfall food. Any sweetened milk (e.g., soy, almond) counts as a pitfall food. Remember: Organic, free-range, or pastured milk doesn't count as a pitfall food. This includes anything made from this healthier source of dairy: ghee, butter, cheese. Conventional dairy and anything made from it counts as a pitfall food.

Q. Which vegetables and whole fruits are pitfall foods?

A. There are only two vegetables that count as pitfall foods: potatoes (all, including sweet potatoes) and corn (when processed into chips; popcorn and corn on the cob are okay). They all give you a quick, addictive rush of serotonin, so they are classified as pitfall foods. Vegetables also have a high-satiety value, so they'll help you feel full. Make sure you're opting for veggies that aren't fried or cooked in a lot of butter or oil. Any fried vegetable counts as a pitfall food.

Q. Which fruits are pitfalls?

A. Any fruit that has not been tampered with is a booster. Fruit can't be dried—grapes are great; raisins are pitfall foods. The fruit has to be pure: no sugar, no oil, no syrup, not juiced, not preserved, not dried, not canned. As long as they're unsweetened, they can be frozen. You can blend whole fruits with skins on into shakes. As a bonus, the skins of apples, pears, plums, and peaches are high in fiber and therefore high on the satiety index.

Q. Do I have to give up alcohol?

A. The 28-day Sugar Brain Fix is not a program designed to treat alcoholism or problem drinking. If you drink, limit drinking to no more than one serving per day for women and two servings per day for men. Alcohol can't be consumed when you're fasting. At any time of the day, count all sugary mixers such as tonic water or juice as a serving of pitfall food. If you're going to drink, favor wine, very-low-carb beers, and liquor mixed with soda water. You can even stretch one serving into two by mixing a half glass of white wine with soda water.

Q. Do I have to give up red meat?

A. No! You can find cuts of high-omega-3 beef—ones that are labeled grass-fed, organic, and/or pasture-raised for a treat. If you can't resist, you can also always have that burger or hot dog at the baseball game. Just count that burger or hot dog as one serving of a pitfall food. Remember that while grass-fed beef has more omega-3s than conventionally raised beef, it still pales in comparison to the potent omega-3 powerhouse of seafood like wild salmon. Grass-fed beef doesn't count as a pitfall, but it also doesn't count as your omega-3 food of the day, either.

Q. I'm on a special diet: diabetic, gluten-free, kosher, for food allergies, vegetarian, vegan, Weight Watchers, . . .

A. No worries. You can still follow the Sugar Brain Fix and simply adhere to the restrictions of points in your program. Check with your health-care professional to see if there are any specific tweaks or considerations you should be aware of when following the Sugar Brain Fix program.

Q. What about salad dressings?

A. I recommend a tablespoon of healthy extra-virgin olive oil (a fantastic staple of the Kediterranean diet) mixed with vinegar (I recommend balsamic, white, red, cider, or champagne vinegars) or freshly squeezed lemon. Remember that most store-bought and restaurant dressings contain huge amounts of sugar and bad fats—which counts as a brain-shrinking pitfall food.

Q. Why don't I have to measure every single calorie?

A. When you're eating vegetables, whole fruits, and good fats, it's much easier to listen to internal cues for physical hunger. You're no longer overwhelmed by the sugar and fat that inundate the pleasure centers in your brain, which leads to overeating and, eventually, a shrunken brain. Thus, it's much easier to eat reasonable portions. The only calorie guideline is for pitfall foods—which is only there to give you a rough guideline on what a serving size entails.

Q. What about diet soda, fruit juice, and artificial sweeteners?

A. Juice—even all-natural fruit juice—has a high concentration of sugar, which floods your brain with serotonin the same way sugar in soda can. Blood sugar spikes, and this can lead to a shrunken brain and expanded waistline. Lemon and lime juice are permitted since they won't spike your blood sugar like other fruit juice. Because of its low sugar content, low-sugar vegetable juice is great. As for diet soda, it may not have calories, but it's linked to weight gain, affects your serotonin levels via your gut, and disrupts metabolism. Lower levels of serotonin can increase cravings for sugar as a means to self-medicate. Additionally, the Kediterranean diet as part of your Sugar Brain Fix helps you to increase the burning of fat for fuel, which requires that blood sugar and insulin levels remain low.

If you need a replacement to wean yourself off diet soda or sugar, look for stevia-sweetened alternatives. Stevia is natural, doesn't disrupt gut bacteria, and won't spike insulin levels.

Q. What about sugar-free gum?

A. Avoid sugar-free gums made with artificial sweeteners. Look for gum made with naturally occurring xylitol instead.

Q. What if I mess up and don't have enough booster foods or booster activities, or have too many pitfalls in one day?

A. You now know that polarized thinking is a pitfall. That means that if you have one day when you mess up, it does *not* mean that your *whole* Sugar Brain Fix is now ruined. Nor should you engage in personalization, another pitfall style of thinking, where one bad day means that *you* are just too weak or a failure.

What you should do is simply move on to the next day. Now maybe you think that you should punish yourself. Perhaps you think if you had four pitfall food servings on day 24 when you were supposed to have only two, having *no* pitfall foods on day 25 is a great way to make up for this.

This cycle of punishment makes things worse. One extreme type of food addiction is binge eating disorder. When a binge eater has binged, the most clinically effective way to deal with the next meal is to eat *as if the binge hadn't happened*. That's right: Even if a binge eater had 2,000 calories at 4 A.M., he or she will actually benefit from going ahead and eating a normal breakfast as opposed to skipping the next two meals to compensate for the binge. The same principle applies to other types of eaters. When you start punishing yourself by compensating, you are affirming a mantra of "I'm bad and need to be punished." In the long run, this sets you up for failure, not success. Just keep following the plan day by day, no matter what you did the day before. If you get off track for multiple days, you can always simply start over at day 1.

Q. What if I relapse after my 28-day Sugar Brain Fix?

A. You may find yourself sneaking three pitfall foods back into your diet, and the following month, you're back up to four. You skip one fasted workout, and the next week, you don't work out at all. You will realize that this puts you back in danger of needing more and more brain-shrinking foods.

Relapse is especially common when you have something difficult or stressful in your life. Use the unexpected tragedies, obstacles, and transitions in your life as an opportunity to be even more diligent in getting what you need through booster activities and brain-boosting foods that will help you to take care of yourself. It's normal to experience sadness and anxiety when going through difficult life incidents, and we all want to feel better when this happens. The only question is: Will you choose unhealthy self-medication through pitfall foods, or will you find healthier ways to take care of your feelings through brain-boosting foods and activities?

IF SOMEONE YOU LOVE IS A FOOD ADDICT . . .

Remember that food addicts get so much negative feedback already in the form of judgment and criticism from themselves and others. What they need is your love and support. The best way to display this is to model healthy behavior and show your support nonverbally by bringing home a healthy meal. Don't make them feel alienated by cooking a "special" meal for them unless they have asked for it. You can benefit the whole family by cooking with booster foods that are good for everyone's health.

When talking to your loved one, move from "you" language to "I" language. So instead of "You really need to lose weight. Are you sure you want to eat that?" say, "I feel really worried about your health. I love you and want to support you. Is there anything I can do?"

Don't enable a food addict by buying pitfall foods at the grocery store. But it's not your responsibility to police them by watching over every bite either. Somewhere in the middle of enabling and policing is supporting, and that's where you want to stay. Remember, the decision to change must ultimately come from them.

Don't be hard on yourself. Just use every relapse as an opportunity that tells you there's still something in your life you are not getting enough of. Perhaps the first time around you felt happier but you still weren't getting the support you needed. Maybe the second time around you can decide to start psychotherapy, hire a trainer, or go to an Overeaters Anonymous meeting for support in addition to all the other healthy rituals that are now a part of your life.

Brain-Boosting Meal Examples

Trying to figure out how to incorporate booster foods into your diet? Let's take a look at an example of a typical day in week 4, when you're cutting your maximum number of pitfall foods per day down to two. In the serotonin-boosting meal example, I'll use a day with no skipped or replaced meals.

To show how you can adjust to the Kediterranean diet template, let's assume the serotonin-boosting meal example is for someone who eats fish, dairy, and eggs—but no meat. In the dopamine example, I'll use a day that includes a replaced breakfast. Let's assume this person is an omnivore. In both examples, I'll exclude water from the meal plans—but you should be drinking water all day long. Being dehydrated can often be mistaken for hunger.

Serotonin-Boosting Meal Example: Remember that the amino acid tryptophan is converted into 5-HTP and then serotonin—with the help of folate, vitamin B_6, vitamin C, zinc, and magnesium. Eating a wide variety of at least seven servings of vegetables and whole fruits daily and healthy sources of protein and fat will ensure you're getting the amino acid, vitamins, and minerals needed for serotonin production. Ensuring you're getting one omega-3-rich food daily increases the brain-boosting benefits. Here's an example.

- **Breakfast:** organic egg omelet (tryptophan, higher omega-3 content than conventional eggs) with spinach (folate), mushrooms (vitamin B_6), and tomatoes (vitamin C); 1/2 cup organic plain yogurt (zinc, higher omega-3 content than conventional dairy); black coffee (magnesium)

- **Lunch:** chilled wild salmon (tryptophan, omega-3-rich food), lentils (folate), chickpeas (zinc), raspberries (vitamin C), slivered almonds (zinc), collard greens salad (magnesium) with olive oil and vinegar dressing (healthy source of good, monounsaturated fat); piece of bread (pitfall food); unsweetened iced tea

- **After Lunch:** black decaf coffee

- **Dinner:** oysters to start (zinc); blackened tempeh (tryptophan) with sesame seeds (magnesium); side of brussels sprouts (folate); bananas (vitamin B_6), strawberries (vitamin C), and ice cream (pitfall food) for dessert; 1 glass of red wine

Fruit and vegetable count (minimum 7): 8
Omega-3-rich food count (minimum 1): 1
Pitfall food count: 2

Dopamine-Boosting Meal Example: Remember that the amino acid tyrosine is converted into L-dopa and then dopamine—with the help of iron, vitamin C, and folate. Eating a wide variety of at least seven servings of vegetables and whole fruits daily and healthy sources of protein and fat will ensure you're getting the amino acid, vitamins, and minerals needed for dopamine production. Ensuring you're getting one omega-3-rich food daily increases the brain-boosting benefits. Here's an example.

- **Breakfast:** beef bone broth made with free-range bones; black coffee with 1 tablespoon virgin coconut oil

- **After Breakfast:** black coffee with stevia

- **Lunch:** walnuts (omega-3-rich food), organic grilled chicken (tyrosine, higher omega-3 content than conventional chicken) over spinach (iron), raspberries (vitamin C), store-bought vinaigrette containing sugar and soybean oil (pitfall food)

- **After Lunch:** hot, unsweetened herbal tea with lemon

- **Dinner:** factory-farmed steak (pitfall food since it's factory-farmed and thus has higher levels of omega-6s); side of brussels sprouts (folate), cauliflower (vitamin C), and swiss chard (folate) sautéed in olive oil (healthy source of good, monounsaturated fat); kiwi (vitamin C) and strawberries (vitamin C) for dessert

Fruit and vegetable count (minimum 7): 7
Omega-3-rich food count (minimum 1): 1
Pitfall food count: 2

Keep Your Pitfalls Manageable

As you choose pitfall foods, be sure that you're choosing manageable servings that won't flood your brain with chemicals and restart your addictions to brain-shrinking foods. If there is something not on this list or if you're not sure what one serving means, then remember that a pitfall food serving contains no more than about 300 calories.

A pitfall food contains a sugar and a bad fat. As a reminder, here's the list of what's considered "sugar" and the list of "bad fats."

Sugar*

- Sugar
- Artificial sweeteners
- Flour
- Fruit juice
- Grains
- Ground corn

*For a complete list of ingredient names, refer to page 196.

Bad Fats

- Anything fried
- Anything in bad oils—which includes all oils except olive (all), virgin coconut, cold- or expeller-pressed canola, walnut, avocado, macadamia nut, and Malaysian palm fruit
- All processed meats, including lunch meat—even white meat
- Conventionally raised/factory-farmed animal products, including meat, milk, eggs, and dairy

1 manageable serving of pitfall food	
2 sausage links	12 saltines or crackers
1 pancake	Small bag of chips
2 tablespoons of maple syrup or artificially flavored syrup	Nuts roasted in an industrial oil
	Dried fruit
1 bagel	Fruit cocktail in syrup
2 tablespoons of nonorganic cream cheese	Small bag of pretzels
	1/2 of a small movie theater popcorn
1 small doughnut	1/2 of a small order of nachos
1 piece of coffee cake	1/2 of a large pretzel
Home fries	Ramen noodles
1 croissant	1/3 box of macaroni and cheese
1 small muffin	8-ounce milk shake
1 biscuit	1 slice of cheesecake
1 slice of pepperoni pizza	1 piece of cake
6 ounces of flavored full-sugar yogurt or artificially sweetened yogurt	1 cup of frozen yogurt
	1 cup of ice cream
1 piece of fried chicken	12 ounces of soda
3 chicken nuggets	12 ounces of diet soda
4-ounce serving of factory-farmed meat	12 ounces of tonic water
Small coleslaw	1 small iced sugary coffee beverage
Small french fries	12 ounces of fruit juice
1 serving of mashed potatoes	2 small cookies
1 baked potato	Small candy bar
1 hot dog	Small milk chocolate bar
2 tablespoons of jelly or jam	6 pieces of licorice
2 ounces of pasta	2 tablespoons of salad dressing that contains sugar or soybean oil
2 factory-farmed meatballs	
Small cheeseburger	2 tablespoons of mayonnaise made with soybean or canola oil that's not expeller-pressed
Tuna or chicken salad in mayonnaise made with soybean oil	
2 pieces of white bread	2 tablespoons of tartar sauce
Large flour tortilla	2 tablespoons of margarine
	2 tablespoons of sugar

Swaps and Switches

One of the best aspects of fixing your sugar brain is how we focus on what we're adding, not on what we're taking away.

You're always going to like certain foods. But with a few simple tweaks, you can get the taste you're craving in a more healthy and sustainable way. As you follow this program, you will actually begin to prefer these booster foods over the pitfall foods they're replacing! I know from my own personal experience. But don't take my word for it. Experience it for yourself.

Instead of this pitfall	Swap with this booster food
coffee with sugar	coffee with 1 tablespoon of virgin coconut oil or organic cream, stevia
orange juice	whole orange
apple juice	whole apple
bacon	grilled organic beef slices
fruit-on-the-bottom yogurt	plain organic yogurt with frozen blueberries
white bread	mashed cauliflower
factory-farmed cream cheese	organic cream cheese
corn flakes or puffed rice cereal	grapefruit
cranberry juice cocktail	sparkling water
diet soda	stevia-sweetened Vitamin Water Zero
soda	unsweetened coffee or tea
tonic water	soda water
Caesar dressing	homemade vinaigrette
ranch dressing	balsamic vinegar
Thousand Island dressing	lemon juice and ground pepper
croutons	sliced red bell peppers
skim milk	organic half-and-half
small cheeseburger	free-range steak
french fries	whole apple slices
egg roll	grilled chicken skewers, organic
spicy tuna roll wrapped with white rice	tuna sashimi, side of edamame
1 cup of white rice	extra steamed vegetables
6-inch cold-cut submarine sandwich on white bread with American cheese and mayonnaise	grilled chicken breast over greens, lots of veggies, extra vinegar, and olive oil
corn chips and salsa	celery and salsa
beef fajitas in flour tortillas	grilled shrimp fajitas in lettuce-leaf wrap
fried chicken	grilled fish
queso	hummus
cream-based soup	broth-based soup
lot of noodles	lots of vegetables
nonorganic beef chili	organic beef, turkey, or veggie chili
potato chips	baby tomatoes

cheddar cheese, nonorganic	cheddar cheese, organic
white pasta	cauliflower rice
mayo with soybean oil	mayo with olive oil
crackers with peanut butter	carrots with hummus
apple pie	frozen whole banana
chocolate milk shake	chocolate pea-protein shake with acai berry
fruit pastry	whole fruit
frozen yogurt with strawberries in syrup	plain yogurt with frozen whole strawberries, stevia
fried	baked, sautéed, grilled, steamed
soybean, corn, peanut oil	mostly olive oil, a little virgin coconut oil

Set Yourself Up for Success

Choosing to commit to something *when you're ready* ensures that this change is coming from the most important place: you. The best predictor for success is your *willingness* to change. When you are truly ready to make a change in your life, then it's time to manifest the health and happiness you've been longing for. All the tools you now have at your disposal will help you to choose foods that help keep your brain healthy.

Goals that are made in public are more likely to be kept than goals made in private. So it's time to go beyond the resolutions you make to yourself in your head—the same resolutions that aren't likely to be kept. Make your journey public. Tell your significant other, a friend, 12-step sponsor, trainer, or health-care professional, and have them sign this contract with you. You'll be making a binding promise to the most important person in this agreement—you. And it's a simple way to keep yourself accountable and get the support you will need on this journey.

Here's your Sugar Brain Fix contract:

I've identified that my pitfall mantra is:

And the mantra that I'd like to have is:

The best thing about having this new mantra will be:

I would rate my willingness to make change on a scale of 0 to 10 (with 0 being not willing to lift a finger and 10 being willing to do whatever it takes):

I, (*your name*) _____ , am committed to following the Sugar Brain Fix for 28 days. I will eat foods that help grow my brain and shrink my waistline while filling my life with booster activities that will change my mantra. Embarking on this journey means that I am affirming my own self-worth, and I am willing to let my behaviors and choices help support this belief.

Signed,   Date:

_____   _____

(You)

_____   _____

(Accountability Buddy: friend, spouse, health-care professional, or sponsor)

Here's where you can journal your own Sugar Brain Fix:

Starting waist measurement ___
Starting weight ___ (or better yet: starting weight with body fat percentage)

In week 1, skip or replace one meal. If you're replacing the meal, write: *bone broth* or *vegan broth* for that meal. If you're skipping it, write: *fasting* next to that meal. In addition to your regular exercise routine, do one fasted workout—just after the skipped or replaced meal.

Day 1, Week 1

Breakfast _____

Lunch _____

Dinner _____

Booster activity _____

Fruit and vegetable count (minimum 7) _____

Omega-3 superfood count (minimum 1) _____

Day 2, Week 1

Breakfast _____

Lunch _____

Dinner _____

Booster activity _____

Fruit and vegetable count (minimum 7) _____

Omega-3 superfood count (minimum 1) _____

Day 3, Week 1

Breakfast _____

Lunch _____

Dinner _____

Booster activity _____

Fruit and vegetable count (minimum 7) _____

Omega-3 superfood count (minimum 1) _____

Day 4, Week 1

Breakfast _____

Lunch _____

Dinner _____

Booster activity _____

Fruit and vegetable count (minimum 7) _____

Omega-3 superfood count (minimum 1) _____

Day 5, Week 1

Breakfast _____

Lunch _____

Dinner _____

Booster activity _____

Fruit and vegetable count (minimum 7) _____

Omega-3 superfood count (minimum 1) _____

Day 6, Week 1

Breakfast _____

Lunch _____

Dinner _____

Booster activity _____

Fruit and vegetable count (minimum 7) _____

Omega-3 superfood count (minimum 1) _____

Day 7, Week 1

Breakfast _____

Lunch _____

Dinner _____

Booster activity _____

Fruit and vegetable count (minimum 7) _____

Omega-3 superfood count (minimum 1) _____

My waistline _____
My weight _____ (or weight and body fat percentage)
What I learned about myself this week was:

_____

_____

_____

What I think I need more of in my life is:

_____

_____

_____

The thing I'm most proud of myself for this week is:

_____

_____

_____

I have noticed the seven pitfall thought patterns (personalization, pervasiveness, paralysis-analysis, pessimism, polarization, psychic, permanence):

Increased _____ Decreased _____ Remained the same _____

I have noticed the seven booster attributes (purpose, peace, pride, power, passion, productivity, pleasure):

Increased _____ Decreased _____ Remained the same _____

Overall, I'm feeling:

_____

_____

_____

_____

_____

In week 2, skip or replace two meals. You can either skip or replace one dinner and the next morning's breakfast, or skip or replace two nonconsecutive meals: one breakfast and one dinner; two breakfasts; or two dinners. If you're replacing the meal, write: *bone broth* or *vegan broth* for that meal. If you're skipping it, write: *fasting* next to that meal. In addition to your regular exercise routine, do at least one fasted workout—just after a skipped or replaced meal. Double your booster activities to two per day.

Day 8, Week 2

Breakfast _____

Lunch _____

Dinner _____

Booster activity 1 _____

Booster activity 2 _____

Fruit and vegetable count (minimum 7) _____

Omega-3 superfood count (minimum 1) _____

Day 9, Week 2

Breakfast _____

Lunch _____

Dinner _____

Booster activity 1 _____

Booster activity 2 _____

Fruit and vegetable count (minimum 7) _____

Omega-3 superfood count (minimum 1) _____

Day 10, Week 2

Breakfast _____

Lunch _____

Dinner _____

Booster activity 1 _____

Booster activity 2 _____

Fruit and vegetable count (minimum 7) _____

Omega-3 superfood count (minimum 1) _____

Day 11, Week 2

Breakfast _____

Lunch _____

Dinner _____

Booster activity 1 _____

Booster activity 2 _____

Fruit and vegetable count (minimum 7) _____

Omega-3 superfood count (minimum 1) _____

Day 12, Week 2

Breakfast _____

Lunch _____

Dinner _____

Booster activity 1 _____

Booster activity 2 _____

Fruit and vegetable count (minimum 7) _____

Omega-3 superfood count (minimum 1) _____

Day 13, Week 2

Breakfast _____

Lunch _____

Dinner _____

Booster activity 1 _____

Booster activity 2 _____

Fruit and vegetable count (minimum 7) _____

Omega-3 superfood count (minimum 1) _____

Day 14, Week 2

Breakfast _____

Lunch _____

Dinner _____

Booster activity 1 _____

Booster activity 2 _____

Fruit and vegetable count (minimum 7) _____

Omega-3 superfood count (minimum 1) _____

My waistline _____
My weight _____ (or weight and body fat percentage)
What I learned about myself this week was:

_____

_____

_____

What I think I need more of in my life is:

_____

_____

_____

The thing I'm most proud of myself for this week is:

_____

_____

_____

I have noticed the seven pitfall thought patterns (personalization, pervasiveness, paralysis-analysis, pessimism, polarization, psychic, permanence):

Increased _____ Decreased _____ Remained the same _____

I have noticed the seven booster attributes (purpose, peace, pride, power, passion, productivity, pleasure):

Increased _____ Decreased _____ Remained the same _____

Overall, I'm feeling:

_____

_____

_____

_____

_____

In week 3, skip or replace three meals. Skip or replace one dinner and the next morning's breakfast plus one additional breakfast or dinner. If this is too difficult, you can skip or replace three nonconsecutive meals: three breakfasts; three dinners; two breakfasts and one dinner; or one breakfast and two dinners. If you're replacing the meal, write: *bone broth* or *vegan broth* for that meal. If you're skipping it, write: *fasting* next to that meal. In addition to your regular exercise routine, do at least two fasted workouts—just after a skipped or replaced meal. Increase your booster activities to three per day.

Day 15, Week 3

Breakfast _____

Lunch _____

Dinner _____

Booster activity 1 _____

Booster activity 2 _____

Booster activity 3 _____

Fruit and vegetable count (minimum 7) _____

Omega-3 superfood count (minimum 1) _____

Pitfall food count (maximum 3) _____

Day 16, Week 3

Breakfast _____

Lunch _____

Dinner _____

Booster activity 1 _____

Booster activity 2 _____

Booster activity 3 _____

Fruit and vegetable count (minimum 7) _____

Omega-3 superfood count (minimum 1) _____

Pitfall food count (maximum 3) _____

Day 17, Week 3

Breakfast _____

Lunch _____

Dinner _____

Booster activity 1 _____

Booster activity 2 _____

Booster activity 3 _____

Fruit and vegetable count (minimum 7) _____

Omega-3 superfood count (minimum 1) _____

Pitfall food count (maximum 3) _____

Day 18, Week 3

Breakfast _____

Lunch _____

Dinner _____

Booster activity 1 _____

Booster activity 2 _____

Booster activity 3 _____

Fruit and vegetable count (minimum 7) _____

Omega-3 superfood count (minimum 1) _____

Pitfall food count (maximum 3) _____

Day 19, Week 3

Breakfast _____

Lunch _____

Dinner _____

Booster activity 1 _____

Booster activity 2 _____

Booster activity 3 _____

Fruit and vegetable count (minimum 7) _____

Omega-3 superfood count (minimum 1) _____

Pitfall food count (maximum 3) _____

Day 20, Week 3

Breakfast _____

Lunch _____

Dinner _____

Booster activity 1 _____

Booster activity 2 _____

Booster activity 3 _____

Fruit and vegetable count (minimum 7) _____

Omega-3 superfood count (minimum 1) _____

Pitfall food count (maximum 3) _____

Day 21, Week 3

Breakfast _____

Lunch _____

Dinner _____

Booster activity 1 _____

Booster activity 2 _____

Booster activity 3 _____

Fruit and vegetable count (minimum 7) _____

Omega-3 superfood count (minimum 1) _____

Pitfall food count (maximum 3) _____

My waistline _____
My weight _____ (or weight and body fat percentage)
What I learned about myself this week was:

_____

_____

_____

What I think I need more of in my life is:

_____

_____

_____

The thing I'm most proud of myself for this week is:

_____

_____

_____

I have noticed the seven pitfall thought patterns (personalization, pervasiveness, paralysis-analysis, pessimism, polarization, psychic, permanence):

Increased _____ Decreased _____ Remained the same _____

I have noticed the seven booster attributes (purpose, peace, pride, power, passion, productivity, pleasure):

Increased _____ Decreased _____ Remained the same _____

Overall, I'm feeling:

_____

_____

_____

_____

_____

In week 4, skip or replace four meals. Skip or replace one dinner and the next morning's breakfast twice this week. Or, skip or replace one dinner and the next morning's breakfast plus two additional nonconsecutive breakfasts or dinners. Or, skip or replace four nonconsecutive meals: four breakfasts; four dinners; or a combination of breakfasts or dinners. If you're replacing the meal, write: *bone broth* or *vegan broth* for that meal. If you're skipping it, write: *fasting* next to that meal. In addition to your regular exercise routine, do at least two fasted workouts—just after the meal you skipped or replaced. Increase your booster activities to four per day.

Day 22, Week 4

Breakfast _____

Lunch _____

Dinner _____

Booster activity 1 _____

Booster activity 2 _____

Booster activity 3 _____

Booster activity 4 _____

Fruit and vegetable count (minimum 7) _____

Omega-3 superfood count (minimum 1) _____

Pitfall food count (maximum 2) _____

Day 23, Week 4

Breakfast _____

Lunch _____

Dinner _____

Booster activity 1 _____

Booster activity 2 _____

Booster activity 3 _____

Booster activity 4 _____

Fruit and vegetable count (minimum 7) _____

Omega-3 superfood count (minimum 1) _____

Pitfall food count (maximum 2) _____

Day 24, Week 4

Breakfast _____

Lunch _____

Dinner _____

Booster activity 1 _____

Booster activity 2 _____

Booster activity 3 _____

Booster activity 4 _____

Fruit and vegetable count (minimum 7) _____

Omega-3 superfood count (minimum 1) _____

Pitfall food count (maximum 2) _____

Day 25, Week 4

Breakfast _____

Lunch _____

Dinner _____

Booster activity 1 _____

Booster activity 2 _____

Booster activity 3 _____

Booster activity 4 _____

Fruit and vegetable count (minimum 7) _____

Omega-3 superfood count (minimum 1) _____

Pitfall food count (maximum 2) _____

Day 26, Week 4

Breakfast _____

Lunch _____

Dinner _____

Booster activity 1 _____

Booster activity 2 _____

Booster activity 3 _____

Booster activity 4 _____

Fruit and vegetable count (minimum 7) _____

Omega-3 superfood count (minimum 1) _____

Pitfall food count (maximum 2) _____

Day 27, Week 4

Breakfast _____

Lunch _____

Dinner _____

Booster activity 1 _____

Booster activity 2 _____

Booster activity 3 _____

Booster activity 4 _____

Fruit and vegetable count (minimum 7) _____

Omega-3 superfood count (minimum 1) _____

Pitfall food count (maximum 2) _____

Day 28, Week 4

Breakfast _____

Lunch _____

Dinner _____

Booster activity 1 _____

Booster activity 2 _____

Booster activity 3 _____

Booster activity 4 _____

Fruit and vegetable count (minimum 7) _____

Omega-3 superfood count (minimum 1) _____

Pitfall food count (maximum 2) _____

My waistline _____
My weight _____ (or weight and body fat percentage)
What I learned about myself this week was:

_____

_____

What I think I need more of in my life is:

_____

_____

The thing I'm most proud of myself for this week is:

_____

_____

What I learned about myself this month was:

_____

_____

The thing I'm most proud of myself for this month is:

_____

_____

I have noticed the seven pitfall thought patterns (personalization, pervasiveness, paralysis-analysis, pessimism, polarization, psychic, permanence):

Increased _____ Decreased _____ Remained the same _____

I have noticed the seven booster attributes (purpose, peace, pride, power, passion, productivity, pleasure):

Increased _____ Decreased _____ Remained the same _____

Overall, I'm feeling:

_____

_____

_____

Congratulations!

Be proud of yourself! You have made it through the 28-day Sugar Brain Fix program. You've reduced or eliminated sugar and bad fats as you've added nourishing foods, intermittent fasting, and fasted workouts to fuel brain growth. You're now following a brain-healthy, belly-fat-busting Kediterranean diet. You have probably figured out by now that my true wish for you is to keep living the principles you have learned here for the rest of your life. And now—through your own experience—you know what it *feels like* to fill your plate, your day, and your life with foods and activities that will keep your brain big and beautiful. I hope you now realize that living this way is not a chore, because feeling good becomes the positive reinforcement that keeps you moving in an upward spiral that can easily last the rest of your life.

My ultimate hope for you is to create so many affirming and boosting relationships, experiences, and activities that food is exactly what it should be: the delicious fuel that helps you live a rich, purpose-filled life. As your waistline continues to shrink and your brain continues to grow, the changes you've made will begin to feel even more rewarding and sustainable.

Here's one final success story to send you on your way.

SUGAR BRAIN FIXED: MELODIE'S STORY

Before starting the Sugar Brain Fix, Melodie had a wake-up call at her doctor's office. When her doctor said she was now almost 190 pounds, she was shocked and saddened. Like so many of people, age and weight can tend to creep up on us. Then one day, you get on a scale as you say to yourself, "How did *that* happen?" Some part of Melodie still considered herself that "that skinny girl" she used to be when she was younger. As Melodie said, "Who was I kidding? I haven't been that girl for over 25 years."

Perhaps the most challenging part for Melodie was that she had *never* dieted or exercised. But with the wake-up call from her doctor, it was clear that it was time for things to change. All the sugar and bad-fat-filled food was shrinking her brain, and the effects of her lifestyle were apparent on the scale. When she heard about my 28-day program, she was all in.

Unlike my family members who were already following a points-based program and exercising fairly regularly, Melodie was going to be changing the way she ate and exercising for the first time in her life. Could she pull it off? Would she be successful in her efforts?

You bet! In fact, I'd say Melodie has made a 180-degree pivot from her old ways.

BEFORE THE SUGAR BRAIN FIX

DATE: 6/18/18
WEIGHT: 189 lbs.
BODY FAT: 92.6 lbs. (49%)
LEAN MASS: 96.3 lbs. (51%)

AFTER THE 28-DAY SUGAR BRAIN FIX +
ONE MONTH OF MAINTENANCE

DATE: 8/17/18
WEIGHT: 175.6 lbs.
BODY FAT: 82.1 lbs. (46.8%)
LEAN MASS: 93.5 lbs. (53.2%)

TOTAL NUMBER OF POUNDS LOST: 13.4
TOTAL NUMBER OF POUNDS OF BODY FAT SHREDDED: 10.5

UPDATE: 2/14/19
WEIGHT: 169.4 lbs.
TOTAL NUMBER OF POUNDS LOST TO DATE: 19.6

THE TAKEAWAY: The Sugar Brain Fix was Melodie's way of paying attention to the wakeup call she was delivered in her doctor's office. Maybe you're someone like Melodie. You've never watched what you ate, fasted, or exercised, and you're scared that the Sugar Brain Fix won't work for you. But if you just start, you can change your brain, body, and life—just like Melodie did.

I checked in with Melodie to see how she was doing and how her life had changed. Here's what she had to say:

- I've stopped drinking soda.

- The flavored creamer in my coffee was hard to give up. Now, I just drink my coffee with half a pack of stevia or just black.

- Before the Sugar Brain Fix, my husband and I would go for ice cream after dinner four to five times a week. We don't do this anymore.

- During the program, I cut out fast food entirely. Now, it's a seldom occasion—maybe once or twice a month.

- I eat lots of booster foods, like avocados and apples.

- I drink lots of water now. I take a water bottle everywhere I go.

- I fast a lot now. My fasts have gotten longer. At least once a week, I'm doing a 20-hour fast with a fasted workout.

- I'm exercising! I think the weight loss and the whole lifestyle change made me able to start a serious exercise program. I went from someone who never exercised to someone who does Orangetheory regularly. Since I have hip and back problems, I have to modify some of the floor exercises. It's hard, but I do it.

APPENDIX A

Sugar Brain–Fixing Recipes

My friend Liana Werner-Gray is the author of *The Earth Diet*, *10-Minute Recipes,* and *Cancer-Free with Food*. The recipes she kindly contributed to this book are free of sugar and bad fats and will help you along your 28-day journey. The only sugars that are used are blueberries, dates, stevia, and monk fruit.

Liana started *The Earth Diet* as a blog in 2009 in an attempt to avoid processed junk foods (full of gluten, dairy, soy, and refined sugars) and live a more natural life. It started when she was faced with declining health and a major wake-up call at just 21 years old. It was then that she decided to change her diet—to find a way to enjoy all her favorite foods but in a healthier, more natural way. We hope the same for you.

Bon appétit!

SOUPS AND BROTHS

HOW TO MAKE A BASIC BONE BROTH

Making bone broth is as simple as placing the bones from a grass-fed animal in a pot or slow cooker, and adding water and apple cider vinegar. The vinegar leaches the minerals out of the bones, which takes at least an hour. It is recommended to cook the bones longer, more like eight hours, to get the most minerals out of them.

If you are pressed for time, you can add some bone broth powder (like Ancient Nutrition Bone Broth Protein Pure) to water and boil that for a superquick recipe.

If bone broth doesn't sound appealing to you, don't force yourself to like it. Some people resonate with it, and others don't. Trust your body, and if you are curious or excited to try it, that is a strong indicator that it would be right for your body. The process for creating a bone broth is:

- Add bones to a Crock-Pot or pot. Add filtered water to fully cover the bones.

- Add apple cider vinegar.

- Add vegetables and bring to a boil, then reduce the heat to low. The skin from the bones will float to the top. Once the broth is cooked, discard.

When making bone broth, you're allowing the collagen to leak out of the bones and form an incredibly nutrient-rich broth that is an anti-inflammatory, helps heal leaky gut, and helps to clear brain fog.

BEEF BONE BROTH WITH ROSEMARY

Total time: 30 minutes prep, 24 hours cooking

Makes 9 cups

Ingredients:

2½ pounds of raw organic grass-fed beef bones

3 tablespoons apple cider vinegar

6 rosemary sprigs

1 teaspoon sea salt

1 teaspoon turmeric

½ teaspoon black pepper

½-inch piece of ginger root, peeled and chopped

1 medium onion, peeled and quartered

2 celery stalks, cut into thirds

2 garlic cloves, smashed

1 tablespoon dried oregano or oregano essential oil

20 cups filtered water

Actions:

Add all the ingredients to a large pot and bring to a boil. Once the liquid is boiling vigorously, lower the heat, cover, and simmer for 24 hours.

Check the broth every few hours and stir.

You will know it's cooked when you poke the bones with a fork and they fall apart and break. When cooked, strain the broth through mesh so you are left with just the liquid. Discard the solids.

Tips:

- You can also put the ingredients into a slow cooker and let the broth cook for 8 to 12 hours.

- Some people like to roast their beef bones before boiling them for a smoky flavor.

- If you store beef broth in the fridge, it will set hard, which is a good sign that the marrow nutrients came out of the bones. It will go to liquid again once heated.

- Store in the fridge for up to 6 days or in the freezer for up to 4 months. If freezing, just allow extra room in the container or jar, as it will expand when frozen.

CHICKEN BONE BROTH

Total time: 30 minutes prep, 24 hours cooking

Makes 9 cups

Ingredients:

Bones from 2 chickens (approx. 2½ pounds of chicken bones)

2 tablespoons apple cider vinegar

1 teaspoon sea salt

1 teaspoon turmeric

½ teaspoon black pepper

½-inch piece of ginger root, peeled and chopped

1 medium onion, peeled and quartered

½ head of broccoli, chopped into chunks

2 celery stalks, cut into thirds

2 carrots, peeled and halved

2 garlic cloves, smashed

1 bay leaf

2 rosemary sprigs

1 tablespoon dried oregano

20 cups filtered water

Actions:

Add all the ingredients to a large pot and bring to a boil. Once the liquid is boiling vigorously, lower the heat, cover, and simmer for 24 hours.

Check the broth every few hours and stir.

You will know it's cooked when you poke the bones with a fork and they fall apart and break. When cooked, strain the broth through mesh so you are left with just the liquid. Discard the solids.

Tips:

- You can also put the ingredients into a slow cooker and let the broth cook for 8 to 12 hours.

- Some people like to roast their chicken bones before boiling them for a smoky flavor. You can also buy two organic rotisserie chickens instead of roasting your own.

- If you store chicken broth in the fridge, it will set hard, which is a good sign that the marrow nutrients came out of the bones. It will go to liquid again once heated.

- Store in the fridge for up to 6 days or in the freezer for up to 4 months. If freezing, just allow extra room in the container or jar, as it will expand when frozen.

VEGETABLE BROTH

Total time: 10 minutes

Makes 4 servings

Ingredients:

4 cups filtered water
1 tablespoon onion powder
1 tablespoon garlic powder
1 tablespoon celery powder
1 tablespoon coriander powder

1 tablespoon fresh parsley
1 tablespoon fresh thyme
2 bay leaves
1 teaspoon sea salt
¼ teaspoon black pepper

Actions:

Place all the ingredients in a large pot over high heat and bring to a boil. Allow to boil for 8 minutes.

When cooled, transfer the broth to an airtight jar or container and store in the fridge or freezer. Unlike a bone broth, vegetable broth will store in the fridge for up to 14 days.

VEGETABLE SOUP

Total time: 10 minutes

Makes 4 servings

Ingredients:

5 cups filtered water
½ teaspoon dried thyme or 1 tablespoon fresh thyme
½ teaspoon dried parsley or 1 tablespoon fresh parsley
½ teaspoon dried oregano
½ teaspoon cumin powder
1 teaspoon sea salt

¼ teaspoon black pepper
½ head of cauliflower
½ head of broccoli
1 carrot
2 celery stalks
Dash of cayenne pepper, optional

Actions:

Place the water, herbs, and spices in a large pot over high heat and bring to a boil. Meanwhile, chop the vegetables into small pieces.

Add the vegetables to the pot and allow the mixture to boil for 7 minutes more. Transfer the soup to bowls and add a dash of cayenne pepper, if desired, for some kick.

IMMUNE-BOOSTING SOUP

Total time: 10 minutes

Makes 2 servings

Ingredients:

1 tablespoon extra-virgin olive oil

1 small yellow onion

8 fresh basil leaves or 1 teaspoon dried basil

1 tablespoon fresh thyme or 1 teaspoon dried thyme

1 tablespoon fresh parsley or 1 teaspoon dried parsley

1 tablespoon fresh cilantro or 1 teaspoon dried coriander

3 fresh sage leaves or 1 teaspoon dried sage

1 teaspoon cumin powder

1 teaspoon turmeric powder

1 teaspoon sea salt

½ teaspoon cracked black pepper

Pinch or 2 of cayenne pepper

1 tablespoon minced garlic

3 medium juice tomatoes

2 cups filtered water

Actions:

Heat the oil in a medium pot over medium heat. Chop the onion and add it to the pot. Cook for 2 minutes until the onion begins to soften. Gather up all your herbs and spices.

When the onion is soft, add the herbs, spices, and garlic and mix well.

Squeeze the tomatoes into the pot. Chop up the tomato skins and add them to the pot as well.

Add the water and let the soup cook for 7 minutes.

Season with more sea salt and pepper, if desired. Top with broccoli sprouts and additional fresh herbs like basil, parsley, and cilantro, if desired.

ENERGY SOUP

Total time: 10 minutes

Makes 2 servings

Ingredients:

1½ cups coconut water or fermented probiotic beverage (kombucha or green tea kombucha)

1 teaspoon dulse flakes

1 to 2 apples, coarsely chopped

1 cup baby spinach leaves

1 green onion

¼ to ½ cup broccoli sprouts, sunflower sprouts, or alfalfa sprouts

1 avocado

Actions:

Blend all the ingredients in a high-powered blender until the mixture is smooth.

Serve the soup topped with fresh herbs like cilantro.

Tips:

- Use a high-powered blender, such as a Vitamix, with a variable-speed dial, to prepare this recipe.

- The soup can be an acquired taste. Tweak the ingredients and amounts to your liking. If you like savory seasonings, add cayenne pepper, garlic, and sea salt to taste.

COCONUT MILK–CHICKEN BROTH THAI SOUP

Total time: 20 minutes

Makes 4 servings

Ingredients:

1 tablespoon virgin coconut oil

2 tablespoons grated fresh ginger

1 tablespoon red or green curry paste

4 cups organic free-range pastured Chicken Bone Broth (page 280)

1 cup Vegetable Broth (page 281)

½ teaspoon sea salt

1 teaspoon amino acids

One 14-ounce can unsweetened coconut milk

2 tablespoons fresh lime juice

1 teaspoon minced lemongrass

¼ cup fresh cilantro, chopped

4 tablespoons broccoli sprouts, chopped

1 cup bean sprouts

Actions:

Heat the oil in a large pot over medium-high heat. Add the ginger and curry paste and cook for 1 minute. Pour in the rest of the ingredients, except for the cilantro, broccoli sprouts, and bean sprouts. Bring to a boil and continue boiling for 8 minutes.

Serve topped with fresh cilantro, broccoli sprouts, and bean sprouts.

Tip:

- Add organic chicken, beef, fish, or shrimp if you want to add protein.

CHICKEN BLACK BEAN NOODLE SOUP

Total time: 15 minutes

Makes 4 servings

Ingredients:

8 ounces organic black bean spaghetti

1 tablespoon virgin coconut oil

2 celery stalks, chopped

1 tablespoon onion powder

1 teaspoon garlic powder

½ teaspoon dried basil

½ teaspoon dried oregano

½ teaspoon dried thyme

¼ teaspoon sea salt

¼ teaspoon pepper

7 cups Chicken Bone Broth (page 280)

1¾ cups Vegetable Broth (page 281) or carton of vegetable broth

½ pound chicken strips

Handful of broccoli sprouts

Actions:

Cook the black bean spaghetti noodles according to the instructions on the package. Drain and set aside.

Place the oil, celery, onion powder, and garlic powder in a large pot over medium-high heat and cook for 1 minute. Pour in the rest of the ingredients, except for the noodles.

Bring to a boil and allow to cook for 7 minutes.

Add the noodles and cook for another minute, until the chicken is cooked through.

Serve topped with broccoli sprouts.

RAW TOMATO SOUP

Total time: 7 minutes

Makes 3 servings

Ingredients:

One 28-ounce can whole tomatoes, in juice

1 rib of celery, roughly chopped

1 cup filtered water

¼ small onion

1 garlic clove

1 teaspoon dried parsley

1 teaspoon dried thyme

1 bay leaf

1 tablespoon fresh lemon juice

¼ teaspoon sea salt

¼ teaspoon black pepper

Actions:

Puree all the ingredients in a blender until smooth.

Taste. Season with more sea salt and pepper, if desired.

Tips:

- For a hot soup, transfer the mixture to a pot. Bring to a boil, then simmer for 7 minutes.

- Serve topped with broccoli sprouts.

KIDNEY BEAN SOUP WITH WATERCRESS AND KALE

Total time: 15 minutes

Makes 4 servings

Ingredients:

1½ tablespoons virgin coconut oil

1 yellow onion, chopped

1 teaspoon garlic powder

3 cups filtered water

1 cup Vegetable Broth (page 281)

Two 15-ounce cans organic kidney beans, drained and rinsed

2 cups kale, diced

2 cups watercress, diced

¼ teaspoon cumin

Black pepper, to taste

Handful of broccoli sprouts

Actions:

Heat the oil in a large saucepan over medium-high heat. Add the onion and garlic powder and cook for 1 ½ minutes.

Add the remaining ingredients and cook for another 12 minutes. Season to taste with cracked black pepper.

Serve topped with broccoli sprouts.

TOMATO, BASIL, AND WHITE BEAN SOUP

Total time: 10 minutes

Makes 4 servings

Ingredients:

1¾ cups Chicken Bone Broth (page 280)

2 teaspoons chili powder

1 teaspoon ground cumin

One 16-ounce can navy beans, drained and rinsed

1 medium chili (your choice of heat), halved and seeded

1 small yellow onion

1 pint grape tomatoes

½ cup fresh basil, plus additional for garnish

¼ cup fresh cilantro

2 tablespoons fresh lime juice

1 tablespoon extra-virgin olive oil

½ teaspoon sea salt

Handful of broccoli sprouts

Actions:

Combine the broth, chili powder, cumin, and beans in a medium pot over medium-high heat.

Meanwhile, place the chili, onion, tomatoes, basil, and cilantro in a food processor and process until smooth.

Transfer the mixture to the pot and boil for 8 minutes. Remove from the heat and stir in the lime juice, olive oil, and sea salt. Garnish with fresh basil and broccoli sprouts.

DELICIOUS LENTIL OREGANO TURMERIC SOUP

Total time: 45 minutes

Makes 4 servings

Ingredients:

5 tablespoons extra-virgin coconut oil

1 yellow onion, chopped

3 garlic cloves, chopped

½-inch piece of ginger, chopped

2 teaspoons cumin

1 teaspoon dried thyme

1 teaspoon sage

1 teaspoon oregano

1 teaspoon turmeric powder

⅛ teaspoon cayenne pepper or more to taste

1 teaspoon sea salt

¼ teaspoon black pepper

6 cups filtered water

1 ½ cups lentils

3 celery stalks, cut into ¼-inch slices

1 cup broccoli sprouts, plus additional for garnish

1 carrot, cut into ¼-inch slices

Juice of 1 lemon

4 tablespoons chopped fresh cilantro

A drizzle of olive oil for each bowl

Actions:

Heat the coconut oil in a large pot and add the onion and garlic. Sauté until golden brown (about 4 minutes). Add the ginger and stir-fry for 1 minute. Add the cumin, thyme, sage, oregano, and turmeric powder and stir-fry for 1 minute more. Add the cayenne pepper, sea salt, and black pepper. Stir-fry for another minute until the spices are fragrant.

Stir in the water, lentils, celery, broccoli sprouts, and carrot. Bring to a boil over high heat, then reduce to medium-low, cover, and simmer for 30 minutes or until the lentils are soft.

Stir in the lemon juice and cilantro. Sprinkle with more sea salt or cayenne pepper to taste. Top each serving with broccoli sprouts and a drizzle of olive oil.

Tip:

- Serve with Gluten-Free Pumpkin Teff Crepes (page 299).

BRAINIAC MUSHROOM SOUP

Total time: 35 minutes

Makes 4 servings

Ingredients:

4 tablespoons virgin coconut oil

2 yellow onions, chopped

1 pound any kind of fresh mushrooms, sliced

4 cups filtered water

2 teaspoons dill

1 tablespoon paprika

1 teaspoon sea salt

1 teaspoon thyme

1 cup unsweetened almond milk

1 tablespoon diatomaceous earth

¼ teaspoon black pepper

2 teaspoons lemon juice (from ½ lemon)

¼ cup fresh parsley, chopped

½ cup vegan sour cream

Squeeze of fresh lemon

Handful of broccoli sprouts

Actions:

Heat the oil in a large pot. Add the onions and sauté for 3 minutes. Add the mushrooms and sauté for another 5 minutes.

Stir in the water, dill, paprika, sea salt, and thyme and continue cooking.

Whisk the almond milk and diatomaceous earth together in a separate bowl. Pour into the soup, stirring well to blend the ingredients. Cover and simmer for 15 minutes, stirring occasionally.

Reduce the heat to low and stir in the pepper, lemon juice, parsley, and sour cream. Mix together and allow to cook for another 5 minutes. Serve topped with broccoli sprouts.

Tips:

- If you want a smoother, less chunky consistency, puree the soup in a blender once it's cooked.

- Serve over cauliflower rice.

GROUNDING VEGETABLE SOUP

Total time: 2 hours

Makes 4 servings

Ingredients:

1 yellow onion	1 tablespoon extra-virgin olive oil
2 large carrots	6 garlic cloves, crushed
2 celery stalks	5 cups filtered water
1 pound pumpkin	½ tablespoon sea salt
½ head of broccoli	1 tablespoon fresh sage or 1 teaspoon dried sage
2 zucchini	Handful of broccoli sprouts

Actions:

Dice the onion, carrots, celery, pumpkin, broccoli, and zucchini into 1-inch cubes and set aside.

Heat the oil in a large saucepan over medium heat. Add the onions, celery, and garlic and sauté until the onions become translucent.

Add the remainder of the diced vegetables to the saucepan, along with the water, sea salt, and sage, and bring to a boil. Simmer over medium heat for 90 minutes, until the vegetables are broken down.

Season with additional sea salt and pepper to taste. Serve topped with broccoli sprouts.

Tip:

- For more protein, add 2 cups dried beans of any kind (soaked for at least 12 hours).

RED TURMERIC CURRY BLACK BEAN NOODLE SOUP WITH BROCCOLI AND BASIL

Total time: 40 minutes

Makes 4 servings

Ingredients:

8 ounces organic black bean spaghetti

1 head of organic broccoli or broccolini, cut into bite-size pieces

1 cup organic snap peas

3 tablespoons olive oil

1 yellow onion, sliced

1 garlic clove, sliced

½-inch piece of fresh ginger, diced

1 teaspoon garlic salt

½ teaspoon black pepper

1 teaspoon red chili flakes

3 tablespoons red curry paste

One 14-ounce can unsweetened coconut milk

2 cups vegetable stock

2 tablespoons MCT oil

1 fresh organic lime, divided

1 small green chili, sliced

1 cup organic bean sprouts

¼ cup fresh organic basil

Actions:

Cook the spaghetti noodles according to the instructions on the package. Drain and set aside.

Steam the broccoli and snap peas and cook until tender. Set aside.

Heat the oil in a pot and add the onion, garlic, and ginger. Stir-fry for 2 to 3 minutes, until the flavors combine and the onion becomes translucent.

Add the garlic salt, pepper, and red chili flakes, and stir-fry for 1 minute.

Add the red curry paste and stir-fry for another minute.

Add the coconut milk, vegetable stock, MCT oil, and half the juice of the lime. Cook over medium-low heat and allow to simmer for 8 minutes so the flavors can combine.

Divide the soup into 4 bowls. Top each serving with noodles, broccoli, snap peas, a sprinkle of red chili flakes, green chili, bean sprouts, basil, and the remaining sliced fresh lime.

CHICKEN NOODLE BONE BROTH SOUP

Total time: 10 minutes

Makes 4 servings

Ingredients:

1 tablespoon coconut oil

2 celery stalks, chopped

1 tablespoon onion powder

1 teaspoon garlic powder

½ teaspoon dried basil

½ teaspoon dried oregano

½ teaspoon dried thyme

¼ teaspoon sea salt

¼ teaspoon pepper

9 cups (72 ounces) Chicken Bone Broth (page 280)

½ pound organic chicken strips

8 ounces shirataki noodles

Actions:

Add the oil, celery, onion powder, and garlic powder to a large pot over medium-high heat. Cook for 2 minutes. Pour in all the remaining ingredients, except for the noodles.

Bring to a boil and allow to cook for 5 minutes.

Add the noodles and cook for another 9 minutes, or until the noodles and chicken are cooked through.

MAINS

GLUTEN-FREE CAULIFLOWER-CRUST "CHEESE" PIZZA

Total time: 40 minutes

Makes 4 servings

Ingredients:

Cauliflower crust

1 medium-size head of cauliflower

2 organic eggs

¼ cup almond flour

¼ cup tigernut flour

¼ cup coconut flour

¼ cup nutritional yeast

¼ teaspoon sea salt

¼ teaspoon black pepper

¼ teaspoon garlic powder

1 teaspoon Italian seasoning

½ teaspoon basil

½ teaspoon oregano

Pizza toppings

⅓ cup sugar-free tomato sauce

¼ cup vegan cheese

½ teaspoon oregano

Handful of fresh basil, for garnish

Actions:

Preheat the oven to 375°F. Line a baking sheet with parchment paper.

Pulse the cauliflower into a fine powder or small rice-shaped pieces in a food processor.

Steam the cauliflower for 5 minutes, until slightly soft. Set aside to cool. When cool, press paper towel or cheesecloth against the cauliflower to absorb as much liquid as possible.

Combine the remaining crust ingredients in a bowl and mix to form a dough. If there's excess liquid, add more flour to ensure the dough isn't too wet. The dough should be dry enough to form and press onto a baking sheet, but not as dry as traditional pizza crust dough.

Shape 1 large crust or 2 small crusts on the prepared baking sheet.

Cook the crust for 10 to 15 minutes, until golden brown. Top with tomato sauce, cheese, and oregano. Cook for 8 minutes or until the cheese is melted. Garnish with fresh basil.

EASY LENTIL LOAF

Total time: 1 hour and 20 minutes

Makes 12 servings

Ingredients:

Coconut oil

8 ounces organic red lentil penne

3 teaspoons flaxseed meal

4 teaspoons filtered water

2 celery stalks, diced

1 large carrot, diced

1 teaspoon onion salt

2 teaspoons garlic salt

2 teaspoons rosemary

3 tablespoons marinara pasta sauce

¼ cup organic tomato sauce

Actions:

Preheat the oven to 350°F. Grease a rectangle cake pan with coconut oil.

Cook the penne according to the instructions on the package. Drain.

Meanwhile, prepare your flax "egg": Combine the flaxseed meal and water in a small bowl. Set aside to thicken.

Place the penne in a food processor or blender. Process until it becomes a thick dough. Transfer to a bowl.

Combine the flax "egg" mixture and all the remaining ingredients, except for the tomato sauce, in a bowl and mix with a wooden spoon until well combined.

Press the mixture into the prepared cake pan and top with an even layer of tomato sauce.

Bake 30 minutes. Remove from the oven and add another layer of tomato sauce. Return to the oven and bake for 30 additional minutes, or until golden brown.

VEGAN BLACK BEAN TACOS

Total time: 45 minutes

Makes 4 servings

Ingredients:

Taco filling

½ cup walnuts

1 cup sundried tomatoes

2 tablespoons extra-virgin olive oil

1 teaspoon dried sage

1 teaspoon fennel seeds

1 teaspoon dried thyme

1 teaspoon dried rosemary

1 teaspoon dried oregano

Pinch of black pepper

Pinch of cayenne pepper

Pinch of salt

1 cup black beans

1 packet coconut meat wraps/tortillas

Toppings

4 tablespoons vegan sour cream

8 tablespoons diced lettuce

1 avocado, sliced

1 tomato, chopped

Handful of vegan "cheese"

Actions:

Preheat the oven to 325°F.

Combine the taco filling ingredients, except for the beans, in a blender. Blend for 5 minutes, until the mixture is moist and sticks together.

Add the beans to the taco filling mixture and use your hands to combine.

Bake for 25 minutes.

Assemble the tacos and serve with your desired toppings.

MEDITERRANEAN OMELET

Total time: 10 minutes

Makes 4 servings

Ingredients:

2 tablespoons extra-virgin olive oil

8 large organic eggs

¼ cup olives, sliced

1 cup spinach

1 small tomato, sliced

Small handful of fresh parsley

1 teaspoon minced garlic

¼ cup organic cheese or nutritional yeast

Pinch of sea salt

Actions:

Heat the oil in a large pan.

Whisk the eggs in a bowl, then pour them into the pan.

As the egg mixture starts to firm up, top it with the olives, spinach, tomato, parsley, garlic, cheese, and salt.

Using a spatula, fold the omelet over in half when the egg mixture is cooked and firm.

CONDIMENTS

HOMEMADE HEMPSEED BUTTER

Total time: 10 minutes

Makes 16 servings

Ingredients:

2 cups hempseeds
4 tablespoons hemp oil
¾ teaspoon sea salt

Actions:

Pulse all the ingredients in a food processor until well combined. Store in a jar and refrigerate.

Tip:

- Add 1 tablespoon cacao for Cacao Hempseed Butter.

SIDES AND SNACKS

WHOLE ROASTED CAULIFLOWER

Total time: 1 hour and 20 minutes

Makes 4 to 6 servings

Ingredients:

2 cups filtered water
½ cup virgin coconut oil
¼ cup lemon juice
2 teaspoons lemon zest
1 teaspoon minced garlic
½ teaspoon ground cumin

¼ teaspoon turmeric
¼ teaspoon black pepper
1 teaspoon dill
¼ teaspoon sea salt
3 tablespoons fresh parsley, diced
1 head of cauliflower

Actions:

Preheat the oven to 350°F. Fill a large baking dish with the water and place on the bottom rack of the oven.

Melt the oil in a saucepan. Mix in all the remaining ingredients, except for the cauliflower.

Place the cauliflower on a separate baking tray or cast-iron skillet and thoroughly cover in the marinade from the saucepan. Cook for 1 hour and 10 minutes.

Tip:

- To brown the cauliflower edges, broil for the last 3 to 5 minutes of cooking.

GLUTEN-FREE PUMPKIN TEFF CREPES

Total time: 10 minutes prep, setting overnight, 10 minutes cooking

Makes 8 crepes

Ingredients:

1 cup teff flour

1 cup unsweetened macadamia nut milk

3 tablespoons filtered water

3 eggs

¼ teaspoon orange zest

1 tablespoon virgin coconut oil, plus more for cooking

2 tablespoons organic canned pumpkin

¼ teaspoon sea salt

Dash of cinnamon

Dash of cardamom

Dash of nutmeg

Actions:

Combine all the ingredients in a blender and process until smooth. Cover and refrigerate the batter overnight.

Heat the oil in a frying pan over medium heat. Pour in ⅛ of the batter. Cook the crepe until it starts to bubble, then flip it over and continue cooking until it's done.

MINI CHOCOLATE SUNFLOWER BUTTER CUPS

Total time: 35 minutes

Makes 12 cups

Ingredients:

¾ cup cacao butter

4 tablespoons cacao powder

½ cup tigernut flour or almond flour

1 tablespoon unsweetened

macadamia nut milk

3 tablespoons monk fruit syrup

13½ teaspoons sunflower butter, unsweetened

Actions:

Melt the cacao butter in a saucepan. Stir in the cacao powder, flour, milk, and syrup.

Spoon 1 teaspoon of the mixture into a baking cup, filling ⅓ of the way. Repeat with the remaining cups. Freeze for 5 minutes.

Remove the cups from the freezer and add 1 teaspoon of sunflower butter to each.

Top the cups with 1 ½ teaspoons of the cacao butter mixture, filling them to the top.

Freeze for 15 minutes to set.

BROCCOLI POPCORN

Total time: 25 minutes

Makes 4 servings

Ingredients:

2 ½ tablespoons extra-virgin olive oil
½ cup nutritional yeast
¾ teaspoon sea salt
1 head of broccoli, chopped into bite-size pieces

Actions:

Preheat the oven to 325°F.

Mix the oil, yeast, and salt thoroughly in a large bowl.

Add the broccoli pieces to the bowl and toss until well coated.

Place the broccoli on a baking sheet and bake for 20 minutes until golden brown and crispy.

Tip:

- Add 1 tablespoon of sesame seeds for extra flavor.

VANILLA PUDDING

Total time: 10 minutes

Makes 4 servings

Ingredients:

1 cup unsweetened vanilla almond milk

1 cup unsweetened coconut milk

1 teaspoon vanilla extract

Dash of sea salt

½ cup chia seeds

1 seedless date, diced

1 fig, diced

Toppings

¼ cup sliced almonds

Handful of walnuts

1 cup blueberries

Actions:

Whisk the almond milk, coconut milk, vanilla, and salt in a bowl until well combined. Stir in the remaining ingredients. Set the pudding in the fridge for 10 minutes.

Transfer the pudding to individual bowls and add toppings.

Tip:

- Leave the pudding in the fridge for an additional 20 minutes to set further if the chia seeds have not gelatinized to your liking.

Variation:

- Use 1 tablespoon of cacao powder for Chocolate Pudding.

COCONUT BACON

Total time: 30 minutes

Makes 3½ cups, 7 servings

Ingredients:

¾ cup apple cider vinegar
¼ cup coconut vinegar
1 tablespoon sea salt
1 tablespoon paprika
2 teaspoons garlic powder

1 teaspoon onion salt
½ teaspoon dried cilantro
½ teaspoon dried parsley
3 cups coconut flakes

Actions:

Preheat the oven to 250°F.

Combine all the ingredients, except the coconut flakes, in a bowl. Mix with a spoon until well combined.

Add the coconut flakes and stir until they're completely coated in the sauce. Let soak for 10 minutes.

Spread the coconut flakes on a baking sheet or other oven-proof dish in a single layer, making sure they are not overlapping.

Bake for 5 to 12 minutes, or until the coconut flakes are crispy and golden brown.

CAULIFLOWER RICE

Total time: 10 minutes

Makes 4 servings

Ingredients:

1 head of cauliflower
1 tablespoon coconut oil
¼ teaspoon sea salt

¼ teaspoon black pepper
¼ teaspoon turmeric powder
¼ teaspoon ginger powder

Actions:

Use a food processor to dice the cauliflower into tiny rice-size pieces.

Heat the oil in a pan, add the cauliflower and spices and sauté for 9 minutes.

Tip:

- Add 1 small diced yellow onion for extra flavor.

BEVERAGES

CHOCOLATE CAULIFLOWER SMOOTHIE

Total time: 10 minutes

Makes 2 servings

Ingredients:

1 tablespoon cacao powder

3 tablespoons hempseeds

2 tablespoons chia seeds

1½ cups unsweetened almond milk

3 seedless dates

1½ cups frozen cauliflower

1 cup frozen blueberries

Dash of salt

Dash of vanilla extract

Actions:

Combine all the ingredients in a high-speed blender and process until smooth.

GOLDEN MILK

Total time: 15 minutes

Makes 2 servings

Ingredients:

3 cups unsweetened coconut milk

1½ teaspoons turmeric powder

Pinch of black pepper

¼ teaspoon ginger powder

¼ teaspoon cinnamon

1 tablespoon MCT coconut oil

Actions:

Add all the ingredients to a saucepan and bring to a boil.

Whisk gently until the mixture is boiling. This will make it creamy.

Serve and enjoy.

THE BIG 3:
BLUEBERRY, BROCCOLI SPROUTS, TURMERIC JUICE

Total time: 10 minutes

Makes 1 serving

Ingredients:

2-inch chunk of turmeric root (or 1 teaspoon dried turmeric powder)

1 cup blueberries

1 cup broccoli sprouts

3 celery stalks

1-inch chunk of ginger

Dash of black pepper

Actions:

Put all the ingredients in a juicer, except for the black pepper.

Juice, sprinkle with black pepper, and drink.

BERRY GREEN JUICE

Total time: 10 minutes

Makes 1 serving

Ingredients:

1 cup blueberries
1 cup blackberries
1 small cucumber
1 large celery stalk

Handful of kale
Handful of fresh cilantro
¼ lemon, peeled
½-inch piece of turmeric

Actions:

Put all the ingredients in a juicer.

Juice and drink.

CELERY JUICE

Total time: 10 minutes

Makes 1 serving

Ingredients:

1 bunch of celery
¼ lemon, peeled

Actions:

Put all the ingredients in a juicer.

Juice and drink.

FLAX MILK

Total time: 5 minutes

Makes 4 servings

Ingredients:

4 cups filtered water

1 cup flaxseeds

Dash of sea salt

¼ teaspoon vanilla extract

Actions:

Put all the ingredients in a blender and mix until a smooth consistency is achieved.

Drain with a cheesecloth or fine mesh strainer to remove any fiber.

CHOCOLATE MILK

Total time: 5 minutes

Makes 4 servings

Ingredients:

1 cup tigernuts (or almonds, macadamia nuts, cashews, or Brazil nuts)

4 cups filtered water

2 seedless dates

Pinch of sea salt

¼ teaspoon vanilla extract

Actions:

Put all the ingredients in a blender.

Mix together until a smooth, milky consistency is achieved.

BRAINIAC GREEN SMOOTHIE

Total time: 5 minutes

Makes 2 servings

Ingredients:

1½ cups unsweetened
almond milk

2 cups kale

1½ cups blueberries

1 cup spinach

¼ cup fresh cilantro

1 cup broccoli sprouts

1 peeled cucumber

Actions:

Put all the ingredients in a blender and mix together until a smooth consistency is achieved.

Tips:

- If you want a smoother mixture, add more water.

- For more creaminess, add 1 peeled avocado.

- For more sweetness, add 3 seedless dates (or 1 packet of stevia).

- For extra protein and vitamins, add 1 tablespoon spirulina.

- Reserve the cucumber skins and use them later as refreshing face wipes.

HOT CHOCOLATE

Total time: 10 minutes

Makes 1 serving

Ingredients:

1 tablespoon cacao powder

1 cup boiling filtered water

1 tablespoon unsweetened
almond milk or coconut milk

1 teaspoon monk fruit or stevia

Actions:

Stir all the ingredients together in a mug and drink.

Variation:

- Add a dash of turmeric and cayenne pepper for Spicy Hot Chocolate.

BRAIN-BOOSTING TURMERIC BLACK PEPPER TEA

Total time: 10 minutes

Makes 1 serving

Ingredients:

2 cups filtered water

1-inch piece of ginger, diced

1 garlic clove, diced

Pinch of cayenne pepper (the beverage should be spicy but comfortable to drink)

¼ teaspoon turmeric powder

Dash of black pepper

1 lemon

Actions:

Place all the ingredients, except for the lemon, in a saucepan and bring to a boil. Reduce the heat to medium and simmer for 7 minutes.

Strain the liquid as you pour it into a teacup.

Squeeze in the juice of the lemon and stir well.

Drink warm.

APPENDIX B

Sugar Brain–Fixing Supplements, Foods, and Practices

Talk to your health-care provider before taking supplements or beginning sauna therapy.

Bone Broth

If you don't have time to make your own broth, bonebroth .com has delicious, organic, and grass-fed broths that have been simmered for 18 to 24 hours. They ship their batches of fresh broth once a week. I've obtained a discount of 10 percent off per order for my readers—use code *drmike*. Bone broth helps me to be successful during my personal weekly fasts.

Curcumin

Curcumin is the active ingredient in the spice turmeric. A 2018 study of subjects with a psychiatric condition associated with low levels of brain-derived neurotrophic factor (BDNF) found that curcumin supplementation increased levels of the growth hormone, which can help you to fix your sugar brain. Whether you consume turmeric in food or take a curcumin supplement, consume it with black pepper/BioPerine and/or fat to enhance its bioavailability.

Gymnema

Gymnema is a plant native to India, Africa, and Australia that contains gymnemic acids. These acids reduce your ability to taste sweet foods, which makes any food containing sugar less appealing. In a 2017 double-blind experiment, subjects ate their favorite candy combined with a placebo lozenge or one made by the company Sweet Defeat containing gymnema. The group that received the Sweet Defeat lozenge reduced their candy intake by 44 percent.

If you are struggling in your transition away from sugar, this supplement could prove to be an effective part of your Sugar Brain Fix. By helping to recalibrate your taste buds away from brain-shrinking foods, it will help to fix your sugar brain.

Infrared Saunas

Changing the composition of your body is one of the best things you can do to reduce toxin exposure, since toxins are stored primarily in fat cells. If you have less body fat, you reduce your capacity to store toxins. The Sugar Brain Fix helps you to shred fat rapidly, which is a wonderful thing. By doing so, you are expelling toxic chemicals from your body. However, these chemicals can potentially be reabsorbed as your body is rapidly shedding fat. Thus, it's important to flush toxins as you're melting fat from your body with the Kediterranean template of the Sugar Brain Fix—since toxins are associated with many diseases.

Anything that helps you sweat will help you get rid of toxins via your skin. Thus, all the exercise you're doing during the Sugar Brain Fix is helpful to achieve a mild detox. For a more robust detoxifying effect, I personally follow the protocol described by George W. Yu, M.D., a researcher involved in detoxifying 9/11 rescue workers and Gulf War vets exposed to toxic debris and chemicals. His protocol combines niacin to mobilize the toxins in your brain and body fat paired with sauna therapy. For the maximum effect, he suggests starting with 50 milligrams niacin (avoid flush-free niacin; the flushing helps with detox) and working your way up to 100 milligrams as you learn to tolerate the flushing effect. Take niacin before you exercise. Then, hop directly in an infrared sauna for 20 to 60 minutes. Finish with a cold shower. All saunas can help you to detoxify via sweat, but infrared saunas are more effective—since infrared can penetrate human tissue deeply and activate sweat glands more effectively than dry saunas. Do this frequently as the fat is coming off rapidly during the 28-day program (e.g., daily). Then, you can go down to two to three times per week after the 28-day program.

I have personally tried several different infrared saunas, and I have found Clearlight Saunas by Jacuzzi to be the highest quality. One concern of infrared saunas is their potentially harmful electromagnetic field (EMF) output. An independent lab looked at the electromagnetic fields of six different infrared saunas. The EMF readings of the other brands ranged from 35 milligauss (mG) to 100 mG; Clearlight's EMF measurement was less than 3 mG. Additionally, these readings are taken directly above the heater in the saunas. Since you're not sitting on the heater, it's reasonable to assume that an EMF of less than 3 mG is reduced to almost 0 mG when sitting on the sauna bench.

Infrared sauna sessions are now widely available in major metropolitan areas for about $30 per session. This, of course, can become costly. Infrared saunas come in different sizes—from compact one-person ones to those that can serve as a hot-yoga room. I've secured a $400–$600 discount and free aromatherapy warmer for my readers by mentioning discount code *drmike*. See their models at infraredsauna.com.

Whole Coffee Fruit Extract

The Sugar Brain Fix program is designed to help you grow your brain and boost BDNF levels. There's one supplement that has a remarkable effect on boosting levels of this growth hormone:

whole coffee fruit extract (WCFE). This ingredient is found in several brain-boosting supplements and may help you to restore a sugar brain back to its former glory.

Omega-3 Superfoods

Research has shown that omega-3s may restore BDNF levels in damaged brains. As you already know, eating omega-3-rich food was associated with having a bigger brain in the landmark sugar brain study. Unfortunately, our polluted world means many seafood sources, the richest sources of both the omega-3 EPA and the omega-3 DHA, contain high levels of mercury and other contaminants. One company I love and trust ships clean, sustainable, and omega-3-rich seafood to your door: Vital Choice. Their website is vitalchoice.com. I've secured a special discount for my readers. Use discount code *drmike* for 10 percent off your first order.

APPENDIX C

Exceptions: Who Should Not Use the Sugar Brain Fix

There are several conditions that the Sugar Brain Fix is not intended to address, and many circumstances in which it should be used only under a health-care professional's supervision. Please read the following section carefully if you have any of the following conditions:

- anorexia or bulimia
- severe depression
- concerns about alcohol or drug use
- obsessive-compulsive disorder (OCD)
- diabetes, on medication, or other health concerns

Anorexia or Bulimia

This book is not for you if you are experiencing anorexia or bulimia. If you're struggling with either one of those conditions, please seek treatment from a health-care professional. These serious eating disorders are characterized by severe self-starvation and a cycle of bingeing and purging, either through self-inflicted vomiting or use of laxatives. The Sugar Brain Fix is not designed to treat these potentially life-threatening eating disorders. Conditions such as anorexia and bulimia can result in serious long-term health problems or even death, so please, if you suspect that you or a loved one is suffering from one of these illnesses, get professional help.

Depression

If you are significantly depressed—feeling helpless, hopeless, frequently crying, often in despair—you need to consult your physician before starting this program. Although the Sugar Brain Fix may be helpful in boosting your mood, first you need to rule out severe depression, which may require the help of a health-care professional.

Drinking or Legal/Illegal Drugs

If you are struggling with an effort to contain your drinking or use of drugs—legal or illegal—you should first seek help with that issue. The Sugar Brain Fix is not a program designed to treat alcohol or drug misuse or addiction.

Obsessive-Compulsive Disorder (OCD)

If you have obsessive thoughts and compulsions related to food, including strict and problematic rituals, this can sometimes be a presentation of obsessive-compulsive disorder (OCD). The Sugar Brain Fix is not a program designed to treat OCD. See a mental health professional for screening and treatment.

Diabetes, on Medication, or Other Health Issues

Finally, if you are on medication, are pregnant or nursing, or have diabetes, gout, GERD, or any other health issues, please check with your health-care professional before starting the Sugar Brain Fix.

BIBLIOGRAPHY

Introduction: Sugar: A Codependent Relationship

Bueno, N. B., et al. "Very-Low-Carbohydrate Ketogenic Diet V. Low-Fat Diet for Long-Term Weight Loss: A Meta-Analysis of Randomised Controlled Trials." *British Journal of Nutrition* 110, no. 7 (2013): 1178–87.

Debette, S., et al. "Visceral Fat Is Associated with Lower Brain Volume in Healthy Middle-Aged Adults." *Annals of Neurology* 68, no. 2 (2010): 136–44.

Guertin, T. L., and A. J. Conger. "Mood and Forbidden Foods' Influence on Perceptions of Binge Eating." *Addictive Behaviors* 24, no. 2 (March 4, 1999): 175–93.

Leibowitz, S. F., and B. G. Hoebel. "Behavioral Neuroscience and Obesity." *The Handbook of Obesity.* Edited by G. Bray, C. Bouchard, and P. James. Marcel Dekker, 2004: 301–71.

Seidelmann, S. B., et al. "Dietary Carbohydrate Intake and Mortality: A Prospective Cohort Study and Meta-Analysis." *The Lancet Public Health* 3, no. 9 (2018): e419–28.

Volkow, N. D., and R. A. Wise. "How Can Drug Addiction Help Us Understand Obesity?" *Nature Neuroscience* 8, no. 5 (2005): 555–60.

Chapter 1. The Evolution of Sugar Brain

Agatston, A. *The South Beach Diet.* Rodale, 2003.

Atkins, R. C. *Dr. Atkins' New Diet Revolution.* M. Evans & Co., 2002.

Avena, N. M., P. Rada, and B. G. Hoebel. "Evidence for Sugar Addiction: Behavioral and Neurochemical Effects of Intermittent, Excessive Sugar Intake." *Neuroscience & Biobehavioral Reviews* 32, no. 1 (2008): 20–39.

D'Adamo, P. J., and C. Whitney. *Eat Right 4 Your Type: The Individualized Diet Solution to Staying Healthy, Living Longer & Achieving Your Ideal Weight.* Putnam, 1996.

DeMaria, E. J., et al. "High Failure Rate after Laparoscopic Adjustable Silicone Gastric Banding for Treatment of Morbid Obesity." *Annals of Surgery* 233, no. 6 (2001): 809–18.

Elkins, G., et al. "Noncompliance with Behavioral Recommendations Following Bariatric Surgery." *Obesity Surgery* 15, no. 4 (2005): 546–51.

Godar, R., et al. "Reduction of High-Fat Diet-Induced Obesity after Chronic Administration of Brain-Derived Neurotrophic Factor in the Hypothalamic Ventromedial Nucleus." *Neuroscience* 194 (2011): 36–52.

Gordon, L. "Global Nutrition Overview: Sugar." Euromonitor International (blog), 2015, blog.euromonitor.com/global-nutrition-overview-sugar.

Hannapel, R., et al. "Postmeal Optogenetic Inhibition of Dorsal or Ventral Hippocampal Pyramidal Neurons Increases Future Intake." *eNeuro* 6, no. 1 (2019).

Harmon, K. "Addicted to Fat: Overeating May Alter the Brain as Much as Hard Drugs." *Scientific American,* March 28, 201).

Harveson, R. M. "History of Sugarbeets." University of Nebraska-Lincoln Institute of Agriculture and Natural Resources CropWatch, 2015, cropwatch.unl.edu/history-sugarbeets.

Jacka, F. N., et al. "Western Diet Is Associated with a Smaller Hippocampus: A Longitudinal Investigation." *BMC Medicine* 13, no. 1 (2015): 215.

Kaufman, F. "The Domino's Effect." *Men's Health*, November 9, 2010.

Kenny, P. J., and P. M. Johnson. "Addiction-Like Reward Dysfunction and Compulsive Eating in Obese Rats: Role for Dopamine D2 Receptors." *Nature Neuroscience* 13 (2010): 635–41.

Lewindon, P. J., L. Harkness, and N. Lewindon. "Randomised Controlled Trial of Sucrose by Mouth for the Relief of Infant Crying after Immunisation." *Archives of Disease in Childhood* 78, no. 5 (1998): 453–56.

Maniam, J., et al. "Sugar Consumption Produces Effects Similar to Early Life Stress Exposure on Hippocampal Markers of Neurogenesis and Stress Response." *Frontiers in Molecular Neuroscience* 8 (2016): 86.

Miller, A. H., and C. L. Raison. "The Role of Inflammation in Depression: From Evolutionary Imperative to Modern Treatment Target." *Nature Reviews Immunology* 16, no. 1 (2016): 22.

Molteni, R., et al. "A High-Fat, Refined Sugar Diet Reduces Hippocampal Brain-Derived Neurotrophic Factor, Neuronal Plasticity, and Learning." *Neuroscience* 112, no. 4 (2002): 803–14.

Richter-Levin, G., and I. Akirav. "Amygdala-Hippocampus Dynamic Interaction in Relation to Memory." *Molecular Neurobiology* 22, no. 1–3 (2000): 11–20.

Rubin, R. D., et al. "The Role of the Hippocampus in Flexible Cognition and Social Behavior." *Frontiers in Human Neuroscience* 8 (2014): 742.

Sapolsky, R. M. "Glucocorticoids and Hippocampal Atrophy in Neuropsychiatric Disorders." *Archives of General Psychiatry* 57, no. 10 (2000): 925–35.

Stice, E., K. S. Burger, and S. Yokum. "Relative Ability of Fat and Sugar Tastes to Activate Reward, Gustatory, and Somatosensory Regions." *American Journal of Clinical Nutrition* 98, no. 6 (2013): 1377–84.

Wang, G. J., et al. "Exposure to Appetitive Food Stimuli Markedly Activates the Human Brain." *NeuroImage* 21, no. 4 (April 2004): 1790–97.

———. "Similarity Between Obesity and Drug Addiction as Assessed by Neuro-functional Imaging: A Concept Review." *Journal of Addictive Diseases* 23, no. 3 (2004): 39–53.

Chapter 2. Willpower Is Not the Problem

Allison, D. B., M. S. Faith, and J. S. Nathan. "Risch's Lambda Values for Human Obesity." *International Journal of Obesity and Related Metabolic Disorders* 20, no. 11, (1996): 990–99.

Arias-Carrión, O., and E. Pöppel. "Dopamine, Learning and Reward-Seeking Behavior." *Acta Neurobiologiae Experimentalis* (Warsaw) 67, no. 4 (2007): 481–88.

Bouchard C., et al. "Inheritance of the Amount and Distribution of Human Body Fat." *International Journal of Obesity* 12, no. 3 (1988): 205–15.

Epel, E. S., et al. "Stress and Body Shape: Stress-Induced Cortisol Secretion Is Consistently Greater Among Women with Central Fat." *Psychosomatic Medicine* 62, no. 5 (September/October 2000): 623–32.

Farooqi, I. S., et al. "Clinical Spectrum of Obesity and Mutations in the Melanocortin 4 Receptor Gene." *New England Journal of Medicine* 348, no. 12 (March 2003): 1085–95.

Lee, J. H., D. R. Reed, and R. A. Price. "Familial Risk Ratios for Extreme Obesity: Implications for Mapping Human Obesity Genes." *International Journal of Obesity and Related Metabolic Disorders* 21, no. 10 (October 1997): 935–40.

Le Magnen, J. "A Role for Opiates in Food Reward and Food Addiction." *Taste, Experience, and Feeding.* Edited by E. D. Capaldi and T. L. Powley. American Psychological Association, 1990.

Li, S., et al. "Physical Activity Attenuates the Genetic Predisposition to Obesity in 20,000 Men and Women from EPIC-Norfolk Prospective Population Study." *PLoS Medicine* 7, no. 10 (2010).

Stice, E., et al. "Obesity, Abnormal Reward Circuitry in Brain Linked: Gene Tied to Dopamine Signaling Also Implicated in Overeating." *ScienceDaily,* October 17, 2008.

Stunkard, A. J., et al. "The Body-Mass Index of Twins Who Have Been Reared Apart." *New England Journal of Medicine* 322, no. 21 (May 24, 1990): 1483–87.

Swift, R. M. "Medications and Alcohol Craving." *Alcohol Research and Health* 23, no. 3 (1999): 207–13.

Tambs, K., et al. "Genetics and Environmental Contributions to the Variance of the Body Mass Index in a Norwegian Sample of First-Degree and Second-Degree Relatives." *American Journal of Human Biology* 3, no. 3 (1991): 257–68.

Vogler, G. P., et al. "Influences of Genes and Shared Family Environment on Adult Body Mass Index Assessed in an Adoption Study by a Comprehensive Path Model." *International Journal of Obesity and Related Metabolic Disorders* 19, no. 1 (January 1995): 40–45.

Wang, G. J., et al. "Brain Dopamine and Obesity." *The Lancet* 357, no. 9253 (2001): 354–57.

Chapter 3. How Food Addiction Fuels Sugar Brain— and Vice Versa

Li, S., et al. "Physical Activity Attenuates the Genetic Predisposition to Obesity in 20,000 Men and Women from EPIC-Norfolk Prospective Population Study." *PLoS Medicine* 7, no. 8 (2010): e1000332.

Payne, C.R., et al. "Internal and External Cues: French and American Explanations for Mindless Eating." *FASEB Journal* 20, no. 4 (2006): A175–76.

Saito, H., et al. "Psychological Factors That Promote Behavior Modification by Obese Patients." *BioPsychoSocial Medicine* 3, no. 1 (2009): 9.

Chapter 4. The Secret of Gradual Detox

Ellis, A., and R. Grieger. *Handbook of Rational-Emotive Therapy.* Springer Publishing, 1977.

Simmons, G. "Are You a Little Low on Serotonin or Dopamine?" *EzineArticles,* December 2007.

Spudich, T. "Cortisol and Weight." *ProjectAware,* January 2007.

Chapter 5. Feeling Anxious: Hungry for Serotonin

Anderson, I. M., et al. "Dieting Reduces Plasma Tryptophan and Alters Brain 5-HT Function in Women." *Psychological Medicine* 20, no. 4 (November 1990): 785–91.

Azad, M. B., et al. "Nonnutritive Sweeteners and Cardiometabolic Health: A Systematic Review and Meta-Analysis of Randomized Controlled Trials and Prospective Cohort Studies." *Canadian Medical Association Journal* 189, no. 28 (2017): E929–E939.

Benwell, M. E., D. J. Balfour, and J. M. Anderson. "Smoking-Associated Changes in the Serotonergic Systems of Discrete Regions of Human Brain." *Psychopharmacology* (Berlin) 102, no. 1 (1990): 68–72.

Bell, C., J. Abrams, and D. Nutt. "Tryptophan Depletion and Its Implications for Psychiatry." *British Journal of Psychiatry* 178, no. 5 (2001): 399–405.

Blanchflower, D. G., A. J. Oswald, and S. Stewart-Brown. "Is Psychological Well-Being Linked to the Consumption of Fruit and Vegetables?" *Social Indicators Research* 114, no. 3 (2013): 785–801.

Blass, E., E. Fitzgerald, and P. Kehoe. "Interactions Between Sucrose, Pain and Isolation Distress." *Pharmacology, Biochemistry and Behavior* 26, no. 3 (March 1987): 483–89.

Denmark, F. L., and M. A. Paludi, eds. *Psychology of Women.* Greenwood Press, 1993.

Formanek, R., and A. Gurian, eds. *Women and Depression: A Lifespan Perspective.* Springer, 1987.

"Get Angry When Hungry? Blame Low Serotonin." *Reuters*, June 30, 2008.

Hoffman, B. M., et al. "Exercise and Pharmacotherapy in Patients with Major Depression: One-Year Follow-up of the SMILE Study." *Psychosomatic Medicine* 73, no. 2 (2011): 127.

Hoffmann, B. R., G. Ronan, and D. Haspula. "The Influence of Sugar and Artificial Sweeteners on Vascular Health during the Onset and Progression of Diabetes." *FASEB Journal* 32, no. 1 supplement (2018): 603–20.

Holt, S. H., J. C. Miller, and P. Petocz. "Interrelationships Among Postprandial Satiety, Glucose and Insulin Responses and Changes in Subsequent Food Intake." *European Journal of Clinical Nutrition* 50, no. 12 (December 1996): 788–97.

Lyubomirsky, S. *The How of Happiness: A New Approach to Getting the Life You Want.* Penguin Press, 2007.

Peciña, S., et al. "Hyperdopaminergic Mutant Mice Have Higher 'Wanting' but Not 'Liking' for Sweet Rewards." *Journal of Neuroscience* 23, no. 28 (October 15, 2003): 9395–402.

Pick, M. "An Introduction to Insulin Resistance." Womentowomen.com, 2004.

Stokes, C., and J. Watson. "Why Lighting Up Always Gets You Down." *Scotland on Sunday*, March 14, 2004.

Suez, J., et al. "Artificial Sweeteners Induce Glucose Intolerance by Altering the Gut Microbiota." *Nature* 514, no. 7521 (2014): 181–86.

Wang, Q. P., et al. "Sucralose Promotes Food Intake through NPY and a Neuronal Fasting Response." *Cell Metabolism* 24, no. 1 (2016): 75–90.

Weissman, M. M., and E. S. Paykel. *The Depressed Woman.* University of Chicago Press, 1974.

Wiley, T. S., and B. Formby, Ph.D. *Lights Out: Sleep, Sugar, and Survival.* Simon & Schuster, 2001.

Wurtman, J. J., Ph.D., and N. F. Marquis, M.D. *The Serotonin Power Diet.* Rodale, 2006.

Yu, W. "A Losing Personality." *Scientific American Mind* 21, no. 6 (January/February 2011): 60–63.

Chapter 6. Feeling Blue: Ravenous for Dopamine

Beckley, J., and H. R. Moskowitz. *Databasing the Consumer Mind: The Crave It!, Drink It!, Buy It! & Healthy You!* Databases. Institute of Food Technologists annual meeting, Anaheim, California, July 2002.

Brain, M., C. W. Bryant, and M. Cunningham. "How Caffeine Works." *Discovery Health*, April 2000.

Dalle G. R., et al. "Personality, Attrition, and Weight Loss in Treatment Seeking Women with Obesity." *Clinical Obesity* 5, no. 5 (2015): 266–72.

Gramling, C. "Gender Gap: Male-Only Gene Affects Men's Dopamine Levels." *Science News* 169, no. 9 (March 1, 2006): 132–33.

Hemat, R. A. S. *Andropathy*. Urotext, 2007.

Johnson, P. M., and P. J. Kenny. "Addiction-Like Reward Dysfunction and Compulsive Eating in Obese Rats: Role for Dopamine D2 Receptors." *Nature Neuroscience* 13, no. 5 (2010): 635–41.

Liau, K. M., et al. "An Open-Label Pilot Study to Assess the Efficacy and Safety of Virgin Coconut Oil in Reducing Visceral Adiposity." *ISRN Pharmacology* (March 2011).

Mumme, K., and W. Stonehouse. "Effects of Medium-Chain Triglycerides on Weight Loss and Body Composition: A Meta-Analysis of Randomized Controlled Trials." *Journal of the Academy of Nutrition and Dietetics* 115, no. 2 (2015): 249–63.

Munro, C., et al. "Sex Differences in Striatal Dopamine Release in Healthy Adults." *Journal of Biological Psychiatry* 58, no. 10 (2006): 966–74.

Redgrave, P., and K. Gurney. "The Short-Latency Dopamine Signal: A Role in Discovering Novel Actions?" *Nature Reviews Neuroscience* 7, no. 12 (December 2006): 967–75.

Schaefer, A. L., et al. "Role of Nutrition in Reducing Antemortem Stress and Meat Quality Aberrations." *Journal of Animal Science* 79, no. suppl_E (2001): E91–E101.

Stice, E., et al. "Relation Between Obesity and Blunted Striatal Response to Food Is Moderated by TaqIA A1 Allele." *Science* 322, no. 5900 (October 17, 2008): 449–52.

Visioli, F., et al. "Dietary Intake of Fish vs. Formulations Leads to Higher Plasma Concentrations of N–3 Fatty Acids." *Lipids* 38, no. 4 (2003): 415–18.

Volnow, N. D. "Evaluating Dopamine Reward Pathway in ADHD: Clinical Implications." *Journal of the American Medical Association* 302, no. 10 (September 9, 2009): 1084–91.

Chapter 7. Feeling Powerless: Starving for Everything

Kabat-Zinn, J. *Wherever You Go, There You Are: Mindfulness Meditation in Everyday Life*. Hyperion, 1994.

Chapter 8. The Secret of Intermittent Fasting

Anson, R. M., et al. "Intermittent Fasting Dissociates Beneficial Effects of Dietary Restriction on Glucose Metabolism and Neuronal Resistance to Injury from Calorie Intake." *Proceedings of the National Academy of Sciences* 100, no. 10 (2003): 6216–20.

Bastani, A., S. Rajabi, and F. Kianimarkani. "The Effects of Fasting During Ramadan on the Concentration of Serotonin, Dopamine, Brain-Derived Neurotrophic Factor and Nerve Growth Factor." *Neurology International* 9, no. 2 (2017): 7043.

Fond, G., et al. "Fasting in Mood Disorders: Neurobiology and Effectiveness. A Review of the Literature." *Psychiatry Research* 209, no. 3 (2013): 253–58.

Harvie, M. N., et al. "The Effects of Intermittent or Continuous Energy Restriction on Weight Loss and Metabolic Disease Risk Markers: A Randomized Trial in Young Overweight Women." *International Journal of Obesity* 35, no. 5 (2011): 714–27.

Imamura, M., et al. "Repeated Thermal Therapy Improves Impaired Vascular Endothelial Function in Patients with Coronary Risk Factors." *Journal of the American College of Cardiology* 38, no. 4 (2001): 1083–88.

Jakubowicz, D., et al. "High Caloric Intake at Breakfast vs. Dinner Differentially Influences Weight Loss of Overweight and Obese Women." *Obesity* 21, no. 12 (2013): 2504–12.

Lee, J., W. Duan, and M. P. Mattson. "Evidence That Brain-Derived Neurotrophic Factor Is Required for Basal Neurogenesis and Mediates, in Part, the Enhancement of Neurogenesis by Dietary Restriction in the Hippocampus of Adult Mice." *Journal of Neurochemistry* 82, no. 6 (2002): 1367–75.

Roseberry, A. G. "Acute Fasting Increases Somatodendritic Dopamine Release in the Ventral Tegmental Area." *Journal of Neurophysiology* 114, no. 2 (2015): 1072–82.

Sievert, K., et al. "Effect of Breakfast on Weight and Energy Intake: Systematic Review and Meta-Analysis of Randomised Controlled Trials." *British Medical Journal* 364 (2019): 142.

Chapter 9. Obsessive Eating: Seeking Security

Huppert, J. D., and D. A. Roth. "Treating Obsessive-Compulsive Disorder with Exposure and Response Prevention." *Behavior Analyst Today* 4, no. 1 (Winter 2003).

Neziroglu, F., and M. Anup. "Relationship of Eating Disorders to OCD." *OCD Chicago,* January 2009.

Schwartz, J. H., and B. Beyette. *Brain Lock: Free Yourself from Obsessive-Compulsive Behavior: A Four-Step Self-Treatment Method to Change Your Brain Chemistry.* ReganBooks, 1996.

Sullivan, S., et al. "Personality Characteristics in Obesity and Relationship with Successful Weight Loss." *International Journal of Obesity* 31, no. 4 (April 1, 2007): 669–74.

Chapter 10. Emotional Eating: The Search for Joy

Albers, S. *50 Ways to Soothe Yourself without Food.* New Harbinger, 2009.

Roth, G. *Breaking Free from Emotional Eating.* Plume, 1993.

Chapter 11. Binge Eating: Regaining Control

Fairburn, C. G. *Overcoming Binge Eating.* Guildford Press, 1995.

Quinlan, K. "Binge Eating Disorder / Compulsive Overeating and Its Treatment." *OCD Center of Los Angeles* (blog), November 16, 2010, https://ocdla.com/binge-eating-compulsive-overeating-treatment-1971.

Chapter 12. Starved for Serotonin: Sugar-Free Ways to Satiate the Craving for Sugar

Albers, S. *50 Ways to Soothe Yourself without Food*. New Harbinger, 2009.

Chapter 13. Dopamine-Deprived: "Kediterranean" Diet–Approved Ways to Satiate the Craving for Fat

Kelly, G. S. "Nutritional and Botanical Interventions to Assist with the Adaptation to Stress." *Alternative Medicine Review* 4, no. 4 (September 1999): 249–65.

Melo, F. H., et al. "Antidepressant-Like Effect of Carvacrol (5-Isopropyl-2-Methylphenol) in Mice: Involvement of Dopaminergic System." *Fundamental & Clinical Pharmacology* 25, no. 3 (June 2011): 362–67.

Schrock, K. "Parsley, Sage, Rosemary and Thyme." *Scientific American Mind*, January/February 2011.

Chapter 14. The Power of Thoughts and Beliefs: Harnessing Your Subconscious to Heal Your Sugar Brain

Kirsch, I. "Hypnotic Enhancement of Cognitive-Behavioral Weight Loss Treatments—Another Meta-Reanalysis." *Journal of Consulting and Clinical Psychology* 64, no. 3 (1996): 517–19.

Appendix B. Sugar Brain–Fixing Supplements

Kumar, P. R., et al. "Omega-3 Fatty Acids Could Alleviate the Risks of Traumatic Brain Injury—A Mini Review." *Journal of Traditional and Complementary Medicine* 4, no. 2 (2014): 89–92.

Reyes-Izquierdo, T., et al. "Modulatory Effect of Coffee Fruit Extract on Plasma Levels of Brain-Derived Neurotrophic Factor in Healthy Subjects." *British Journal of Nutrition* 110, no. 3 (2013): 420–25.

Stice, E., S. Yokum, and J. M. Gau. "Gymnemic Acids Lozenge Reduces Short-Term Consumption of High-Sugar Food: A Placebo Controlled Experiment." *Journal of Psychopharmacology* 31, no. 11 (2017): 1496–1502.

Wynn, J. K., et al. "The Effects of Curcumin on Brain-Derived Neurotrophic Factor and Cognition in Schizophrenia: A Randomized Controlled Study." *Schizophrenia Research* 195 (2018): 572–73.

INDEX

Note: Page numbers in *italics* indicate recipes, and page numbers in parentheses indicate noncontiguous references.

B

emotional eating and, 156–157
Mediterranean diet and, xi–xii
shrinking. *See* brain, shrinking from
  sugar and bad fats; hippocampus;
  sugar brain
tolerance dangers, 26–27, 33–34
Brain-Boosting Turmeric Black Pepper
  Tea, *308*

brain chemistry. *See also* dopamine *references*; serotonin *references*
  binge eating and, 167, 168, 169, 170,
    171, 172
  boosters and, 49–50
  emotional eating and, 159–160
  feeling hunger and, 39–40
  feeling out of control and, 117–124
  fine-tuning, 56–57
  food addiction proof, 19–21
  gradual detox, new habits and, 47–48
  keeping in balance, 22–24
  medication for addictions and, 34–35
  pitfall activities and, 48
  Sugar Brain Fix addressing, 29
  thought patterns and, 25–26,
    108–109
  why typical diets don't work and,
    26–28
  withdrawal from addiction and,
    35–36 (*See also* gradual detox)
  yo-yo dieting and, 36–37
brain-derived neurotropic factor (BDNF)
  diet creating more, xii, xiii–xiv
  fasted workouts boosting, 38, 47, 49,
    51, 128
  ketosis boosting levels, xiii
  omega-3s and restoring, 312
  sugar depleting, 7
  supplement boosting, 311–312
  weight loss and, 7
  what it is and does, xii
The Brain Fog Fix (Dow), xii

brain, growing
  BDNF and, 38, 47, 49, 128, 159–160
    (*See also* brain-derived neurotropic
    factor (BDNF))
  boosters and, 49, 175, 220, 235–236
    (*See also* booster activities; booster
    qualities)
  emotions in perspective and, 165

intermittent fasting and, 125, 132
journaling and, 240
olive oil and, 101
omega-3s and, 103, 104
Sugar Brain Fix and, 8, 26, 27, 38, 51,
  74, 235–236 (*See also* Sugar Brain
  Fix program guide)
waistline shrinking and, xiii
whole fruits and, 8
brain, shrinking from sugar and bad fats.
  See also hippocampus; sugar brain
  about: overview of, xii
  amygdala and, 13, 14, 15, 40, 156
  dopamine levels and, 22
  factory-farmed meats and, xiii
  feelings/symptoms of, 12–13, 50–51
  historical perspective, 5
  hypothalamus and, 13–14, 15, 40,
    159, 188
  memory, addiction and, 12–16
  other carbs shrinking brain and, 7–8
  research showing, 6–7
  reversing, xiii, 128
  standard American diet and, 5
Brainiac Green Smoothie, *306–307*
Brainiac Mushroom Soup, *289*
Brianne's story, 181–183
broccoli and broccoli sprouts
  about: nutrients in, 191, 203
  The Big 3: Blueberry Broccoli Sprouts
    Turmeric Juice, *304*
  Broccoli Popcorn, *300*
  Grounding Vegetable Soup, *290*
  other recipes with, *280–281, 283,
    284, 285, 288, 306–307*
  Red Turmeric Curry Black Bean Noo-
    dle Soup with Broccoli and Basil,
    291
  Vegetable Soup, *281–282*
bulimia, 313

C

caffeine, viii, 33–34, 90–91, 107–109,
  111–112, 115
calories, not counting, 243
canola oil, 102
Carol's story (author's mom), 57–59
cauliflower
  about: nutrients in, 191, 203; as

Index

H

habits, healthy new. *See also* booster qualities; gradual detox; mantras *references*; pitfall thought patterns, reframing; Sugar Brain Fix program guide
  about: overview of creating, 47–48
  time to establish in brain, 47
happiness at your discretion, 85
health issues, Sugar Brain Fix and, 313–314
heart, conversation with, 122–123
hemp seed butter, homemade, *297*
hippocampus
  addiction to sugar and, 13–16
  BDNF growing, 128
  emotional eating and, 156–157
  healthy, effects of, 15, 236
  memory, triggers, food consumption and, 14–15, 156
  shrinking from sugar and bad fats, 6, 12–13, 15
Homemade Hemp Seed Butter, *297*
Hot Chocolate, *307*
hunger
  Americans vs. French, 40
  getting to know, 38–40
  insulin levels and, 74–76
  intermittent fasting and, 39–40, 75
  noticing how you feel, 39
  noticing when you feel, 38
  riding the wave of, 174
  tolerance of feelings triggering, 39–40
  typical time cycle for, 39
hypnosis. *See* self-hypnosis
hypothalamus, 13–14, 15, 40, 159, 188

I

Immune-Boosting Soup, *282*
impulsive, feeling, 12–13
inflammation
  brain-boosting foods reducing, 235–236
  depression and, 12–13
  Mediterranean diet reducing, xii
  omega-3s compared to omega-6s and, 11, 104
  omega-3s to reduce. *See* omega-3s

  sugar brain and, 13, 97
  Sugar Brain Fix and, 49, 51
infrared saunas, 310–311
insulin resistance, 74–76, 126
intermittent fasting, 125–133
  benefits of, 125–128
  boosting serotonin levels, 127
  exceptions precaution, 132
  fluids during, 131
  hunger cycle and, 39–40, 75
  meal structure during, 128–131
  schedule during Sugar Brain Fix, 128–131, 237, 238–239
  skipping meals, 125–126, 127
  week 1, 128–130
  week 2, 130
  week 3, 130
  week 4, 130–131

J

Jenna's story, 167–171, 176
Jennifer's story, 139–140, 153
journal
  about: overview of structure and purpose, 240
  setting yourself up for success, 252–253
  week 1, 254–257
  week 2, 258–261
  week 3, 262–266
  week 4, 267–271
joy, search for. *See* emotional eating
juices. *See* recipes, beverages

K

kale and spinach
  about: nutrients in, 191, 203
  Berry Green Juice, *305*
  Brainiac Green Smoothie, *306–307*
  Kidney Bean Soup with Watercress and Kale, *286–287*
Kediterranean diet. *See also* recipes *references*; Sugar Brain Fix program guide
  advantages of, 126
  bypassing side effects of keto diet, xiv–xv
  flexibility of, xvi

329

ABOUT THE AUTHOR

Dr. Mike Dow, Psy.D., Ph.D., is *New York Times* best-selling author and is America's go-to therapist.

As a brain health, mental health, relationship, and addiction expert, Dr. Mike has hosted hit shows on several networks. He is currently a host for Disney+. Additionally, Dr. Mike was the co-host of E!'s *Sex with Brody*, VH1's *Couples Therapy*, ID's *My Strange Criminal Addiction*, LOGO's *That Sex Show*, and TLC's *Freaky Eaters*, and *My 600-lb Life Reunion*. In addition, Mike was the network spokesperson for TLC's *My Strange Addiction*.

He is part of Dr. Oz's core team of experts, a recurring guest co-host on *The Doctors*, and has made regular appearances on *Today*, *Rachael Ray*, *Wendy Williams*, *Meredith Vieira*, *Ricki Lake*, *Nancy Grace*, and *Dr. Drew on Call*. You've also seen him as the therapist to the Housewives on Bravo's *The Real Housewives of Orange County*, Tyler and Catelynn's therapist on MTV's *Teen Mom*, LaToya Jackson's therapist on OWN's *My Life with LaToya*, and the Bachelor's therapist on Freeform's *Ben and Lauren*.

Dr. Mike began his career working with the Los Angeles Department of Mental Health before transitioning to private practice. He has an M.S. in Marriage and Family Therapy, a Psy.D. in Psychology, and a Ph.D. in Clinical Sexology. He practices adult and child psychotherapy, couples therapy, family therapy, sex therapy, and hypnotherapy. Dr. Mike is a graduate of USC, where he was a Presidential Scholar.

Website: drmikedow.com

Hay House Titles of Related Interest

YOU CAN HEAL YOUR LIFE, *the movie,* starring Louise Hay & Friends
(available as a 1-DVD program, an expanded 2-DVD set,
and an online streaming video)
Learn more at www.hayhouse.com/louise-movie

THE SHIFT, *the movie,*starring Dr. Wayne W. Dyer
(available as a 1-DVD program, an expanded 2-DVD set,
and an online streaming video)
Learn more at www.hayhouse.com/the-shift-movie

***

CANCER-FREE WITH FOOD: *A Step-by-Step Plan with 100+ Recipes to Fight
Disease, Nourish Your Body & Restore Your Health,* by Liana Werner-Gray

COMPLETE KETO: *A Guide to Transforming Your Body and Your Mind for
Life,* by Drew Manning

MEDICAL MEDIUM LIFE-CHANGING FOODS: *Save Yourself and the Ones
You Love with the Hidden Healing Powers of Fruits & Vegetables,*
by Anthony William

SUPER FUEL: *Ketogenic Keys to Unlock the Secrets of Good Fats, Bad Fats,
and Great Health,* by Dr. James DiNicolantonio and Dr. Joseph Mercola

All of the above are available at your local bookstore,
or may be ordered by contacting Hay House (see next page).

***

We hope you enjoyed this Hay House book. If you'd like to receive our online catalog featuring additional information on Hay House books and products, or if you'd like to find out more about the Hay Foundation, please contact:

Hay House, Inc., P.O. Box 5100, Carlsbad, CA 92018-5100
(760) 431-7695 or (800) 654-5126
(760) 431-6948 (fax) or (800) 650-5115 (fax)
www.hayhouse.com® • www.hayfoundation.org

———

Published in Australia by: Hay House Australia Pty. Ltd.,
18/36 Ralph St., Alexandria NSW 2015
Phone: 612-9669-4299 • *Fax:* 612-9669-4144
www.hayhouse.com.au

Published in the United Kingdom by: Hay House UK, Ltd.,
The Sixth Floor, Watson House, 54 Baker Street, London W1U 7BU
Phone: +44 (0)20 3927 7290 • *Fax:* +44 (0)20 3927 7291
www.hayhouse.co.uk

Published in India by: Hay House Publishers India,
Muskaan Complex, Plot No. 3, B-2, Vasant Kunj, New Delhi 110 070
Phone: 91-11-4176-1620 • *Fax:* 91-11-4176-1630
www.hayhouse.co.in

———

Access New Knowledge.
Anytime. Anywhere.

Learn and evolve at your own pace
with the world's leading experts.